S0-FSO-784

Wednesday Night at the Lab:
Antibiotics, Bioengineering, Contraceptives, Drugs and Ethics

edited by
Kenneth L. Rinehart, Jr.
William O. McClure
Theodore L. Brown
University of Illinois

HARPER & ROW, PUBLISHERS
NEW YORK, EVANSTON, SAN FRANCISCO, LONDON

WEDNESDAY NIGHT AT THE LAB:
Antibiotics, Bioengineering, Contraceptives, Drugs and Ethics

Copyright © 1973 by University of Illinois

Printed in the United States of America. All rights reserved. No part of this book may be used or reproduced in any manner whatsoever without written permission except in the case of brief quotations embodied in critical articles and reviews. For information address Harper & Row, Publishers, Inc., 10 East 53rd Street, New York, N.Y. 10022.

Standard Book Number: 06–045409–1

Library of Congress Catalog Card Number: 73–281

CONTENTS

PREFACE

After decades of accepting unquestioningly the virtues of science and of spending billions in funding research, the public of late has begun to ask, rather loudly, whether the benefits of the new technology outweigh its costs to the environment, whether genetic engineering violates higher ethical principles, and whether science offers any hopeful solution to the Malthusian specter of overpopulation. It is not easy for the public to find answers to these and similar questions, and it usually must choose between the facile generalities of the popular press and the hard technicalities of science textbooks. In the present book, thirteen research scientists from universities and industry attempt to answer some of the questions posed by current science by discussing, in nontechnical language, present directions in our own fields and the relevance of those fields to the problems of modern society. We hope that what we have written will help put science in context, both for students in introductory courses and for the general public, whose normal exposure to science is through the popular press.

The series of lectures on which this book is based had its inception in May 1970, when, following the U.S. invasion of Cambodia and the deaths of students at Kent State University, the National Guard was ringing our campus at the University of Illinois for the second time that spring. Although classes continued to meet, alternative paths of communication among students and faculty were explored, including a daily afternoon discussion period. In those informal meetings a number of the students argued that the material covered in classes had very little relationship to the problems of the world. Accordingly, a "Relevant Chemistry" series was proposed in an attempt to clarify the role of chemistry, both in causing some of the major problems of ecology, environment, and health, and in solving them.

In the fall of 1970 we arranged a series of nine lectures, on successive Wednesday nights, by speakers from our Departments of Chemistry and Biochemistry, from other departments on campus, and from outside the university. The series continued with more lectures in the spring of 1971, and with four each in the fall of 1971 and spring of 1972. Thus, although our campus crisis was the stimulus for the program, the series ran successfully long after the crisis was past.

Each speaker was asked to discuss a current problem, including the chemical basis for the problem or its solution. He was requested to assume that his audience would consist of students and townspeople with no more than an elementary background in science. Response was enthusiastic, our large lecture hall in Noyes Laboratory was often filled to overflowing, and spirited discussion followed most of the lectures. The series apparently satisfied a need felt by both groups for communication between nonspecialists and specialists in the sciences. Tapes were made of all the lectures in order to allow broadcasts later on the University's radio station.

A cohesive group of the lectures was chosen to be transcribed, and these were revised by the authors into appropriate form for publication in this book. We have endeavored here to maintain the informal tone of the original presentations.

We wish to thank the other members of the "Wednesday Night at the Lab" Committee, who were students (Alan and Kathy Muirhead, Hugh Parkhurst, Craig Miller, Bill Pearson, Tod Brethauer, Marty Watson) and faculty (Jack Hudson, Bob Lowstuter, John Lombardi, Dave Natusch, John Wood, Arnold Hartley, John Quinn) in the School of Chemical Sciences, for their invaluable efforts in planning and supporting the lectures. It is our belief that the "Wednesday Night at the Lab" experiment has been a success, and we anticipate that it will be continued. To that end, royalties from this book will be used by the School of Chemical Sciences to help support the program in the future.

Urbana, Illinois   *Kenneth L. Rinehart, Jr.*
                                                     William O. McClure
                                                     Theodore L. Brown

ABOUT THE AUTHORS

John E. Baldwin, Ph.D., is Professor of Chemistry at the University of Oregon, Eugene, where he and his students carry out research on the mechanisms of organic chemical reactions. He is a member of the President's Science Advisory Committee.

Theodore L. Brown, Ph.D., is Professor of Chemistry at the University of Illinois, Urbana—Champaign. His research interests are mainly in the area of physical-inorganic and organometallic chemistry.

Barry Commoner, Ph.D., is Professor of Botany at Washington University, St. Louis, Mo., and Director of the Center for the Biology of Natural Systems. He is well known for his writing and lecturing activities on matters of environmental concern. His most recent book, The Closing Circle, was published in 1971 by Knopf, New York.

Carl Djerassi, Ph.D., is Professor of Chemistry, Stanford University, Stanford, Calif., President of Syntex Research, and Chairman of the Board of Directors of Zoecon Corporation. He is well known for his research accomplishments in natural products chemistry and in mass spectrometry.

William G. Huber, Ph.D., is Professor of Veterinary Pharmacology at the University of Illinois, Urbana—Champaign. His research activities are concerned mainly with veterinary pharmacology and antibiotic residues in meat.

Julius E. Johnson, Ph.D., is Vice President and Director of Research and Development, Dow Chemical Company, Midland, Mich. Dr. Johnson is a biochemist whose research interests include toxicology and the effects of herbicides, fungicides, insecticides, and nematocides.

John R. Lombardi, Ph.D., is Assistant Professor of Chemistry at the University of Illinois, Urbana—Champaign. His research activities lie in the area of chemical physics.

William O. McClure, Ph.D., is Assistant Professor of Biochemistry at the University of Illinois, Urbana—Champaign. His research activities are centered on the study of proteins of the central and peripheral nervous system.

Robert L. Metcalf, Ph.D., is Professor of Zoology, Entomology, and Agricultural Entomology at the University of Illinois, Urbana—Champaign. He has been actively investigating the environmental fates of pesticides and industrial chemicals and has recently developed a class of biodegradable insecticides.

Phillip S. Myers, Ph.D., is Professor of Mechanical Engineering, University of Wisconsin, Madison, and a former president of the Society of Automotive Engineers. His research interests include the study of combustion in automobile engines.

Kenneth L. Rinehart, Jr., Ph.D., is Professor of Chemistry at the University of Illinois, Urbana–Champaign. He has devoted a major fraction of his research activity to the isolation, structural characterization, and modification of antibiotics.

Robert L. Sinsheimer, Ph.D., is Chairman of the Division of Biology at the California Institute of Technology, Pasadena. His research interests lie in the area of molecular biology, and include studies of nucleic acids and bacterial viruses.

Robert L. Switzer, Ph.D., is Assistant Professor of Biochemistry at the University of Illinois, Urbana–Champaign. He is interested in the study of enzymes and the regulation of enzyme activity in metabolism.

INTRODUCTION

While applauding this series of issue-oriented popular forums sponsored by the George C. Miller Lectures and the School of Chemical Sciences at the University of Illinois, the nagging hope that lingers is that the theme will be caught up by others so that many more people will listen and learn.

We have come a long way these past several years in the realization that continuous and predictable economic growth is no longer sufficient in itself. The tradition of our country has been that growth is a good thing, and it has developed quite naturally that as our population has increased we have built on the necessity of economic growth to maintain a decent life. That growth has been based for the most part on the exploitation of our natural resources, the production of goods and their quick consumption in what has been a seemingly perpetual cycle that allows for no lag in the economy. Yet as our numbers have increased, as our resources have diminished, as our environment has eroded, many counter thoughts have developed. There is a present desire to look at economic growth without assuming, as we traditionally have, that whatever promotes it is good. The lectures included in this series touch on various aspects of that change and force us to consider how our society can learn to substitute other interests, ideas or services for those things which have long dominated our economic design. The contribution they make may, in fact, be of fundamental importance, for they leave one with the idea that until such substitutes are developed, a drastic change in our system might prove dangerous to the nation's social foundation.

Although the authors treat seriously with a category of problems under the headings The Environment, The Environment and Life, Life, and Politics, they do not suggest a moratorium on the use of science and technology but rather recognize that the growing anxiety to hold on to what we have could depress innovation and creativity and make us unwilling to gamble on something better. Instead, they heighten human vitality and push the desire for a more useful expression of the human spirit which I believe must be preserved as the very essence of civilized progress. It is through such frank public discussion and examination that we will come to understand that the momentous risks ahead call on us to take policy steps to guide our economic machine rather than allow the eventual exhaustion of our physical assets to do it for us.

Science and technology cannot always be represented as the immediate or even ultimate solution to all our public problems. Yet they have become such a part of our culture that we look to them to suggest ways of solving our problems by their positive employment in a manner consonant with our traditional democratic concepts. Their better utilization requires a number of forums: the professional community, the Congress, the executive departments and agencies of government, the courts, the special interest groups, and the public at large. Since the public forum not only has the greatest influence of all these but is perhaps the one most likely to respond to emotional stimuli, we recognize the need for an improved public grasp of technology. These lectures have recognized that, for they give the feeling of having evolved out of a town-meeting-like confrontation where the opportunity to gradually and constantly educate the public is a fundamental goal. As we attempt to find solutions to the major dilemmas facing our civilization, the ability to enlist the help of more and improved science and technology may well depend on our having achieved that objective.

Better decision making through an improved process of a public education and choice could very well have been the theme for this series. None of the authors has come late upon the scene. Despite the fact that the technical community and the public employ rather different criteria of importance concerning technical problems and issues, each of them has played some part in narrowing the communications gap. Gathering them together under one bill of fare is precisely the kind of effort and good will that is needed to move us all closer together.

When we consider that there is often a long time lag between the moment when a technological innovation is first brought into commercial use and the time when its secondary effects are recognized as being seriously adverse, we must realize how important it is to understand each other. As a technological society, we tend to operate on the basis of a short time span. If a product is marketable and appealing, the public wants it in quantity and wants it now. On the other hand, when the unwanted side effects become evident, that same public often insists on quick correction. The lecturers in this series prod us to look ahead and to be less bitter about the errors that are still bound to occur. Each of them helps to sort out troublesome issues and to present them in a rational way even though some of them are problems which have become deeply ingrained in the fabric of everyday life. They give strength to the idea that it may be possible after all to learn how to handle such problems in a rational and democratic way. In offering this possibility, they do not pretend to foresee or identify all aspects of scientific and technological innovation or to lead us unfailingly down the preferred technical paths.

What we are left with is that the choice is ultimately the public's. Since that is where we want it to be, these lectures sustain the idea that we need not be pessimistic about our ability to do better.

Hartford, Connecticut   *Emilio Q. Daddario*

THE ENVIRONMENTAL COST OF ECONOMIC GROWTH[1]

Barry Commoner

INTRODUCTION

This paper is concerned with an evaluation of the environmental costs of economic growth in the United States. This is a complex issue which has appeared rather suddenly on the horizon of public affairs; it therefore suffers somewhat from a high ratio of concern to fact. In addition, the issue is one which happens not to coincide with the domain of any established academic discipline. For environmental costs have been, until rather recently, so far removed from the concerns of orthodox economics as to have been nearly banished from that realm under the term "externalities." And for its part, the discipline of ecology has, also until very recently, maintained a position of lofty disdain for such mundane matters as the price of ecological purity.

It is useful to begin with a brief summary of the ecological background of the issue.

1. The environment is a system comprising the earth's living things and the thin global skin of air, water and soil which is their habitat.

2. This system, the ecosphere, is the product of the joint, interdigitated evolution of living things and of the physical and chemical

[1] A similar article under this title appears in *Energy, Economic Growth, and Environment*, S. H. Schurr, *ed*, Baltimore, Johns Hopkins University Press, 1972, Chap. 2.

constituents of the earth's surface. On the time scale of human life the evolutionary development of the ecosphere has been very slow and irreversible. Hence the ecosphere is irreplaceable; if the system should be destroyed, it could never be reconstituted or replaced either by natural processes or by human effort.

3. The basic functional element of the ecosphere is the ecological cycle, in which each separate element influences the behavior of the rest of the cycle, and is in turn itself influenced by it. For example, in surface waters fish excrete organic waste, which is converted by bacteria to inorganic products; in turn, the latter are nutrients for algal growth; the algae are eaten by the fish, and the cycle is complete. Such a cyclical process accomplishes the self-purification of the environmental system, in that wastes produced in one step in the cycle become the necessary raw materials for the next step. Such cycles are cybernetically self-governed, dynamically maintaining a steady state condition of indefinite duration. However if sufficiently stressed by an external agency, such a cycle may exceed the limits of its self-governing processes and eventually collapse. Thus, if the water cycle is overloaded with organic animal waste, the amount of oxygen needed to support waste decomposition by the bacteria of decay may be greater than the oxygen available in the water. The oxygen level is then reduced to zero. Lacking the needed oxygen, the bacteria die and this phase of the cycle stops, halting the cycle as a whole. It becomes evident, then, that there is an inherent limit to the turnover rate of local ecosystems and of the global ecosystem as a whole.

4. Human beings are dependent on the ecosphere not only for their biological requirements (oxygen, water, food) but also for resources which are essential to all their productive activities. These resources, together with underground minerals, are the irreplaceable and essential foundation of all human activities.

5. If we regard economic processes as the means which govern the disposition and use of resources available to human society, then it is evident from the above that the continued availability of those resources which are derived from the ecosphere (non-mineral resources), and therefore the stability of the ecosystem, is an essential prerequisite for the success of any economic system. More bluntly, any economic system which hopes to survive must be compatible with the continued operation of the ecosystem.

6. Because the turnover rate of an ecosystem is inherently limited, there is a corresponding limit to the rate of production of any of its constituents. Different segments of the global ecosystem (soil, fresh water, marine ecosystems) operate at different intrinsic turnover rates and therefore differ in the limits of their productivity. On purely

theoretical grounds it is self-evident that any economic system which is impelled, by its own requirements for stability, to grow by constantly increasing the rate at which it extracts wealth from the ecosystem must eventually drive the ecosystem to a state of collapse. Computation of the rate limits of the global ecosystem or of any major part of it are, as yet, in a rather primitive state. Apart from the foregoing theoretical and as yet unspecified limit to economic growth, such a limit may arise much more rapidly if the growth of the economic system is dependent on productive activities which are especially destructive of the stability of the ecosystem.

7. Unlike all other forms of life, human beings are capable of exerting environmental effects which extend, both quantitatively and qualitatively, far beyond their influence as biological organisms. Human activities have also introduced into the environment not only intense stresses due to natural agents (such as bodily wastes), but also wholly new substances not encountered in natural environmental processes: artificial radioisotopes, detergents, pesticides, plastics, a variety of toxic metals and gases, and a host of man-made, synthetic substances. These human intrusions on the natural environment have thrown major segments of the ecosystem out of balance. Environmental pollution is the symptom of the resultant breakdown of the environmental cycles.

THE PROBLEM

In order to evaluate the cost of economic growth in terms of the resultant environmental deterioration, it is, of course, necessary to define both terms, if possible in quantitative dimensions that might permit a description of their relationship. The common definition of economic growth would appear to be applicable here: the increase in the goods generated by economic activity. Environmental deterioration is a more elusive concept. On the basis of the foregoing discussion it may be defined as degradative changes in the ecosystems which are the habitat of all life on the planet. The problem is, then, to describe such ecological changes in terms that can be related, quantitatively if possible, to the processes of economic growth—to increased production of economic goods.

To begin, we can take note of the self-governing nature of the ecosystem. It is this property which ensures its stability and continued activity. This basic property helps to define both the process of ecological degradation and the nature of the agencies that can induce it. We can define ecological, or environmental, degradation as a process which so stresses an ecosystem as to reduce its capability for self-adjustment, and which, therefore, if continued, can impose an irreversible stress on the system and cause it to collapse.

An agency which is capable of exerting such an effect on an ecosystem must arise from *outside* that system. This results from the cyclical nature of the ecosystem, which brings about, automatically, the system's readjustment to any internal change in the number or activity of any of its normal biological constituents. For what characterizes the behavior of a constituent which is part of an ecological cycle is that it both influences and is influenced by the remainder of the cycle. For example, organic waste produced by fish in a closed aquatic ecosystem, such as a balanced aquarium, cannot degrade the system because the waste is converted to algal nutrients, and simply moves through the ecological cycle back to fish. In contrast, if organic waste intrudes upon this same ecosystem from without, it is certain to speed up the cycle's turnover rate, and if sufficiently intense, to consume all of the available oxygen, and bring the cycle to a halt.

The internal changes in an ecosystem which occur in response to an external stress are complex, nonlinear processes and not readily reduced to simple quantitative indices. The aquatic ecosystem is one of the relatively few instances in which this goal can, to some degree, be approached—in that oxygen tension is a sensitive internal indicator of the system's approach to instability. However, in most cases such internal measures of the state of an ecosystem have not yet been elucidated. Hence, as a practical, but, it is to be hoped, temporary expedient we need to fall back on a measure of the *impact* on the ecosystem of an external degradative agency as an index of environmental quality. This expedient has the virtue of enabling the quantitative comparison of the effects of ecological impacts of different origins, a matter of particular importance in connection with their relation to economic processes. Such data can later be translated to the resultant internal changes, when the necessary ecological information becomes available.

In what follows, then, the environmental cost of a given economic process will be represented by its *environmental impact,* a term which has the dimensions of the amount of an agency external to the ecosystem which, by intruding upon it, tends to degrade the system's capacity for self-adjustment.

Turning now to the possible environmental impacts that may result from *human* activity, we find the situation somewhat complicated by the special role of human beings on the earth. In one sense, human beings are simply another animal in the earth's ecosystem, consuming oxygen and organic foodstuff and producing carbon dioxide, organic wastes, heat, and more people. In this role, the human being is a constituent part of an ecosystem and therefore in terms of the previous definition exerts no environmental impact on it. However, a human population has a zero environmental impact only as long as it is in fact part of an eco-system, which is the case, for example, if food is acquired from soil which receives the population's organic waste. If a population is separated from this cycle, for example by settling in a city their wastes are intruded, with or without treatment, into surface waters. Now the population is no longer a part of the soil ecosystem, and the wastes become *external* to the aquatic system on which they intrude. Here an environmental impact is generated, leading to water pollution.

On the basis of these considerations, then, people—viewed simply as biological organisms—generate an environmental impact only insofar as they become separated from the ecosystem to which, in nature, terrestrial animals belong. This is, of course, nearly universally true in the United States. The intensity of this environmental impact is generally proportional to the population size.

All other environmental impacts are generated not by human bio-logical activities, but by human *productive activities*, and are therefore governed by economic processes. Such impacts may be generated in several different ways:

1. Certain economic gains can be derived from an ecosystem by exploiting its biological productivity. In these cases, a constituent of the ecosystem which has economic value—for example, an agricultur-al crop, timber or fish—is withdrawn from the ecosystem. Insofar as the withdrawn substance or a suitable substitute fails to return as nutrient to the ecosystem from which it was removed it constitutes a drain on that system which cannot continue indefinitely without causing it to collapse. Destructive erosion of the soil following excessive exploita-tion, or the incipient destruction of the whaling industry due to the extinction of whales are examples of such effects.

2. Environmental stress may also arise from an intrusion of oppo-site sign to that described above—that is the amount of some component of the ecosystem is augmented from outside that system. This may be done either for the purpose of disposing of waste or in order to acceler-ate the system's rate of turnover and thus increase its yield. Examples of these effects are the intrusion of sewage into surface water, and the intensive use of fertilizer nitrogen in agriculture. In the latter case, following a reduction in the nitrogen available from the soil's natural store of nutrient (its organic humus) due to a period of over-exploitation through uncompensated crop withdrawal (a stress of the type described in paragraph 1, above) the nitrate level is artificially raised by adding fertilizer to the soil's ecological cycle. Because of the low efficiency

of nutrient uptake by the crop's roots, (which is in turn a result of in-adequate soil oxygen due to reduced porposity stemming from the de-creased humus content) a considerable portion of the fertilizer leaches from the soil into surface waters, where it becomes an external stress on the aquatic ecosystem, causing algal overgrowths and the resulting breakdown of the self-purifying aquatic cycle.

3. Apart from the above stresses—which represent the impact of externally altered concentrations of natural ecosystem constituents—environmental impact may be due to the intrusion into an ecosystem of a substance wholly foreign to it. Thus, DDT has a powerful environmental impact in part because it readily upsets the naturally balanced ecological relations among insect pests, the plants they attack, and the insects which, in turn, prey on the pests. DDT-induced outbreaks of insect pests often result. In general, there is a considerable risk of environmental pollution whenever productive activity introduces substances which are foreign to the natural environment.

We turn now to the practical problem of evaluating the environmental cost of economic growth. The most general theoretical aspect of this problem has already been alluded to. Given that the global eco-system is closed, and that its integrity is essential to the continued operation of any conceivable economic system, it is evident that there must be an upper limit to the growth of productive activities on the earth.

However, such a theoretical statement is hardly an effective guide to practice. The chief reason is that the theory fails to specify the time scale in which the ecological limitation on economic growth is likely to take effect. For one can readily grant the truth of such an abstract theorem—for example, that economic growth will eventually be limited by the extinction of the sun—and disregard its practical consequences because of the rather long time scale involved, in this case some billions of years.

Accordingly it would seem useful to make the problem more concrete by examining the relationship between economic growth and environmental impact in the real world. And since growth is, of course, a time-dependent process, this suggests the value of an historical approach.

THE ORIGINS OF ENVIRONMENTAL IMPACT

In what follows, I wish to report the results of an initial effort to describe the origins of environmental impacts in the United States. Most United States pollution problems are of relatively recent origin.

The post-war period, 1945–46, is a convenient benchmark, for a number of pollutants—man-made radioisotopes, detergents, plastics, synthetic pesticides and herbicides—are due to the emergence, after the war, of new productive technologies. The statistical data available for this period in the United States provide a useful opportunity to compare the changes in the levels of various pollutants with the concurrent activities of the United States productive system that might be related to their environmental effects.[2]

Although, unfortunately, we lack sufficient comprehensive data on the actual environmental levels of most pollutants in the United States, some estimates of historical changes can be made from intermittent observations, and from computed data on emissions of pollutants from their sources. Some of the available data are summarized in Table 1, which indicates that since 1946, emissions of pollutants have increased by 200 to 2000 per cent. In the case of phosphate, which is a pollutant of surface waters, and enters mainly from municipal sewage, data on the long term trends are available. In the 30-year period between 1910 and 1940, phosphorus output from municipal sewage increased gradually from about 17 million lb. per year to about 40 million lb. per year. Thereafter the rate of output rose rapidly; so that in the 30-year period 1940 to 1970 phosphorus output increased to about 300 million lb. per year.

It should be noted that these are data regarding the computed *emission* of pollutants, which are not necessarily descriptive of their actual concentrations in the environment or of their ultimate effects on the ecosystems or on human health. Numerous, complex and inter-related processes intervene between the entry of a pollutant into the ecosystem and the expression of its biological effect. Moreover, two or more pollutants may interact synergistically to intensify the separate effects. Most of these processes are still too poorly understood to enable us to convert the amount of a pollutant entering an ecosystem to a quantitative estimate of its degradative effects. Nevertheless it is evident that these effects (such as the incidence of respiratory disease due to air pollutants, or of algal overgrowths due to phosphate and nitrate) have increased sharply, along with the rapid rise of pollutant levels, since 1946. Since pollutant emission is a direct measure of the activity of the source, it is a useful way to estimate the contributions of different sources to the overall degradation of the environment.

---

[2]This study has been carried out as part of the program of the American Association for the Advancement of Science Committee on Environmental Alterations in collaberation with Michael Corr and Paul J. Stamler. For a preliminary report of this work, see Commoner, B., Corr, M., and Stamler, P. J., Environment 13:3, 2 (1971).

TABLE 1
Post-War Increases In Pollutant Emissions

| Pollutant | Annual Production | | | | Per cent Increase Over Indicated Period |
	Year	Amount	Year	Amount	
Inorganic Fertilizer Nitrogen	1949	$.91 \times 10^6$ tons	1968	6.8×10^6 tons	648
Synthetic Organic Pesticides	1950	286×10^6 lb.	1967	1050×10^6 lb.	267
Detergent Phosphorus	1946	11×10^6 lb.	1968	214×10^6 lb.	1,845
Tetraethyl Lead[2]	1946	$.048 \times 10^6$ tons	1967	$.25 \times 10^6$ tons	415
Nitrogen Oxides[2]	1946	10.6^1	1947	77.5^1	630
Beer Bottles	1950	6.5×10^6 gross	1967	45.5×10^6 gross	595

[1]Dimension = NOx (ppm) × gasoline consumption (gals × 10^{-6}); estimated from product of passenger vehicle gasoline consumption and ppm of NOx emitted by engines of average compression ratio 5.9 (1946) and 9.5 (1967) under running conditions, at 15 in. manifold pressure. NOx emitted: 500 ppm in 1946; 1200 ppm in 1967.
[2]Automotive emissions.

If we define the amount of a given pollutant introduced annually into the environment as the *environmental impact* (I), it then becomes possible to relate this value to the effects of three major factors that might influence the value of I by means of the following identity:

$$I = \text{Population} \quad \frac{\text{Economic Good}}{\text{Population}} \quad \frac{\text{Pollutant}}{\text{Economic Good}}$$

Here **Population** refers to the size of the United States population in a given year, **Economic Good** refers to the amount of a designated good produced (or where appropriate, consumed) during the given year, and **Pollutant** refers to the amount of a specific pollutant (defined as above) released into the environment as a result of the production (or consumption) of the designated good, during the given year. This relationship enables the estimation of the contribution of three factors to the total environmental impact: (a) the size of the population; (b) production (or consumption) per capita, ("affluence"); (c) the environmental impact (amount of pollutant) generated per unit of production (or consumption), which reflects the nature of the productive technology.

Since we are concerned with identifying the sources of the sharp increases in the environmental impacts experienced in the United States in the period 1946 to the present, it is of interest to examine the

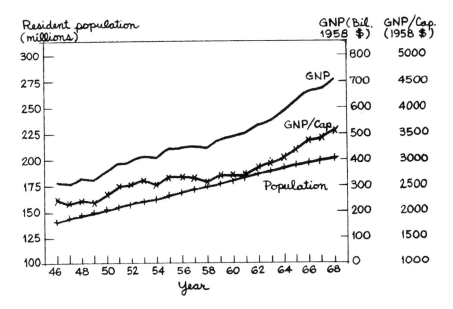

Figure 1:   Changes in populations, Gross National Product (GNP; reduced to 1958 dollars) and GNP per capita for the United States since 1946.   Data are from Department of Commerce, Statistical Abstract of the United States, U. S. Government Printing Office, Washington, D. C. 1970, p. 5 and Department of Commerce, The National Income and Product Accounts of the United States 1929-1965, U. S. Government Printing Office, Washington, D. C. 1966, pp. 4-5.

concurrent changes in the nation's productive activities.   The most general data relevant to these changes are presented in Figure 1. In the period 1946 to 1968 United States population has increased, at an approximately constant rate, by about 42 per cent; GNP (adjusted to 1958 dollars) has increased exponentially by about 126 per cent in that period; GNP per capita has also increased approximately exponentially by about 59 per cent.

We can see at once that, as a first approximation, the contribution of population growth to the overall values of the environmental impacts generated since 1946 is of the order of 40 per cent. In most cases, this represents a relatively small contribution to the total environmental impact, since as indicated in Table I, these values increased by 200 to 2000 per cent, in that period of time.

In order to evaluate the effects of the remaining factors it is useful to examine the growth rates of different sectors of the productive economy. For this purpose a series of productive activities which are likely to contribute significantly to environmental impact and are representative of the overall pattern of the economy have been selected. From the annual production (or, where appropriate, consumption) data for the United States as a whole, which are available from government statistical reports, the annual percentage rates of increase or decrease are calculated, by computer. From results of these computations it is possible to derive certain useful generalizations about the pattern of economic growth, which are relevant to environmental impacts, in the United States.

1. Production and consumption of certain goods have increased at an annual rate about equal to the annual rate of increase of the population so that *per capita* production remains essentially unchanged. This group includes food, fabric and clothing, major household appliances, and certain basic metals and building materials, including steel, copper, and brick. In effect, with respect to these basic items average affluence—per capita production (or consumption)—has remained essentially unchanged in the period 1946-1968.

2. The annual production of certain goods has decreased since 1946, or has increased at an annual rate below that of the population. Horsepower produced by work animals is the extreme case; it declined at an annual rate of about 10 per cent. Other items in this category are: saponifiable fat, cotton fiber, wool fiber, lumber, milk, railroad horsepower, and railroad freight. These are goods which have been significantly displaced in the pattern of production during the course of the overall growth of the economy. Cultivated farm acreage also declined in this period.

3. Among the productive activities which have increased at an annual rate in excess of that exhibited by the population, the following classes can be discerned:

A. Certain of the rapidly increasing productive activities are substitutes for activities that have declined in rate, relative to population. These generally represent technological displacement of an older process by a newer one, with the sum of goods produced remaining essentially constant, per capita, or increasing somewhat. These displacement processes include the following: natural fibers (cotton and wool) by synthetic fibers; lumber by plastics; soap by detergents; steel by aluminum and cement; railroad freight by truck freight; harvested acreage by fertilizer; returnable by nonreturnable bottles.

B. Certain of the rapidly growing productive activities evident in the data are secondary consequences of displacement processes. Thus the displacement of natural products by synthetic ones involves the use of increased amounts of synthetic organic chemicals, so that this category has increased sharply. Moreover, since many organic syntheses require chlorine as a reagent, the rate of chlorine production has also increased rapidly. Finally, because chlorine is efficiently produced in a mercury electrolytic cell, the use of mercury for this purpose has also increased at a very considerable rate. Similarly, the rapidly rising rate of power utilization is, in part, a secondary consequence of certain displacement processes, for a number of the new technologies are more power-consumptive than the technologies which they replace.

C. Finally, among the rapidly growing productive activities are some which represent neither displacements of older technologies, nor sequelae to such displacements, but true increments in per capita availability of goods. An example of this category is consumer electronics (radios, television sets, sound equipment, etc.). Such items represent true increases in affluence.

In sum, the pattern of growth in the United States economy in the period 1946-1968 may be generalized as follows. Basic life necessities, representing perhaps one-third of the total GNP, have grown in annual production at about the pace of population growth, so that no significant overall change in *per capita* production has taken place in this period. However, within these general categories of goods—food, fiber and clothing, freight haulage, household necessities—there has been a pronounced displacement of natural products by synthetic ones, of power-conservative products by relatively power-consumptive ones, of reusable containers by disposable ones.

THE ENVIRONMENTAL IMPACT OF ECONOMIC GROWTH

Given the foregoing conclusions we can now rephrase the original question. What are the relative costs, in intensity of environmental impact, of the several distinctive features of the growth of the United States economy from 1946 to the present? Reasonably complete quantitative answers to this question are, unfortunately, well beyond the present state of knowledge. At the present time it is possible in most cases to provide only an informal, qualitative, description of the changes in environmental impact which have been induced by the post-war transformation of the United States economy. In some cases it is also possible to produce a quantitative evaluation in the form of an Environmental Impact Index and in a few cases a partial Environmental Impact Inventory can be constructed. As shown below, such evidence leads to the general conclusion that in most of the technological displacements which have accompanied the growth of the United States economy since 1946, *the new technology has an appreciably greater environmental impact than the technology which it has displaced, and that the post-war technological transformation of productive activities is the chief reason for the present environmental crisis.*

Agricultural Production

As shown in Figure 2 agricultural production in the United States, as measured by the U. S. Department of Agriculture Crop Index, has increased at about the same rate as the population since 1946. However, the technological methods for achieving agricultural production have changed significantly in that period. One important change is illustrated by Figure 2, which shows that although agricultural production per capita has increased only slightly, harvested acreage has decreased, and the use of inorganic nitrogen fertilizer has risen sharply. This displacement process—of fertilizer for land—leads to a considerably increased environmental impact.

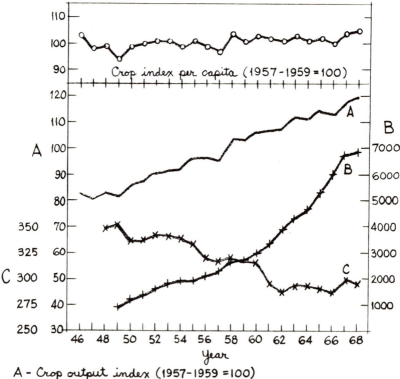

A - Crop output index (1957-1959 =100)
B - Fertilizer nitrogen (1000's of tons)
C - Millions of acres harvested

Figure 2: Changes in total crop output (as determined by U.S.D.A. Crop Index), in crop output per capita, in harvested acreage, and in annual use of inorganic nitrogen fertilizer in the United States since 1946. Data are from Agricultural Statistics, U. S. Government Printing Office, Washington, D. C., 1967, pp. 531, 544, 583; 1970, pp. 444, 454, 481.

Briefly stated the relevant ecological situation is the following. Nitrogen, an essential constituent of all living things, is available to plants in nature from organic nitrogen, stored in the soil in the form of humus. Humus is broken down by bacteria to release inorganic forms of nitrogen, eventually as nitrate. The latter is taken up by the plant roots and reconverted to organic matter, such as the plant's protein. Finally the plant may be eaten by a grazing animal, which returns to the soil as bodily wastes the nitrogen not retained in the growth of its own body.

Agriculture imposes a negative drain on this cycle; nitrogen is removed from the system in the form of the plant crop or of the livestock produced from it. In ecologically sound husbandry all of the organic nitrogen produced by the soil system, other than the food itself—plant residues, manure, garbage—is returned to the soil, where it converted by microbial processes to humus and thus helps to restore the soil's organic nitrogen content. The deficit, if it is not too large, can be made up by the process of nitrogen fixation—in which bacteria, usually in close association with the roots of certain plants, take up nitrogen gas from the air and convert it into organic form. If the nitrogen cycle is not in balance, agriculture "mines" the soil nitrogen, progressively depleting it. This process does more than reduce the store of organic nitrogen available to support plant growth, for humus is not only a nutrient store. Due to its polymeric structure humus is also responsible for the porosity of the soil to air. And air is essential to the soil, not only as a source of nitrogen for fixation, but also because its oxygen is essential to the root's metabolic activity, which in turn is the driving force for the absorption of nutrients by the roots. In the United States, for example in corn belt soils, about one-half of the original soil organic nitrogen has been lost since 1880. Naturally, other things being equal, such soil is relatively infertile and produces relatively poor crop yields. However, beginning after World War II a technological solution was intensively applied to this problem: sharply increasing amounts of inorganic nitrogen were applied to the soil in the form of fertilizer. Annual nitrogen fertilizer usage in the United States increased by an order of magnitude in 1946-1968.

In effect, then, nitrogen fertilizer can be regarded as a substitute for land. With the intensive use of fertilizer it becomes possible to accelerate the turnover rate of the soil ecosystem, so that each acre of soil annually produces more food than before. The economic benefits of this new agricultural technology are appreciable, and self-evident. However, this economic advantage may be counterbalanced by the increased impact on the environment. This arises because, given the reduced humus content of the soil, the plant's roots do not efficiently absorb the added fertilizer. As a result an appreciable part leaches from the soil as nitrate and enters surface waters where it becomes a serious pollutant. Nitrate may encourage algal overgrowths, which in their inevitable death and decay tend to break down the self-purifying aquatic cycle.

Excess nitrate from fertilizer drainage leads to another environmental impact, which may affect human health. While nitrate in food and drinking water appears to be relatively innocuous, *nitrite* is not. Nitrite combines with hemoglobin in the blood, converting it to methemoglobin—which cannot carry oxygen. Unfortunately nitrate can be converted to nitrite by the action of bacteria in the intestinal tract, especially in infants, causing asphyxiation and even death. On these grounds, the United States Public Health Service has established 10 ppm of nitrate nitrogen as the acceptable limit of nitrate in drinking water. In a number of agricultural areas in the United States nitrate levels in water supplies obtained from wells, and in some instances from surface waters have exceeded this limit. Our own studies in the area of Decatur, Illinois show quite directly that in the spring of 1970 when the city's water supply, which is derived from an impoundment of the Sangamon River, recorded 9 ppm of nitrate nitrogen, a minimum of 60 per cent of the nitrate was derived from inorganic fertilizer applied to the surrounding farmland.

The effect of this change in agricultural technology is evident from Table 2, which compares the influence of the several relevant factors

TABLE 2
Environmental Impact Index

	Index Factors			Total Index $(a \times b \times c)$ Fertilizer Nitrogen (1000's of tons)
	a	*b*	*c*	
	Population (1000's)	Crop Production Population (Prod. units/cap.)	Fertilizer Nitrogen Crop Production (tons/prod. unit)	
1949	149,304	5.43×10^{-7}	11,284[1]	914
1968	199,846	6.00×10^{-7}	57,008	6841
1968:1949	1.34	1.11	5.05	7.48
Increase, %	34	11	405	648

[1] The crop output index is an indicator of agricultural productivity with the 1957-1959 average = 100.

on the total environmental impact due to fertilizer nitrogen in 1949 and 1968. During that period the total annual use of fertilizer nitrogen, the total environmental impact, increased 648 per cent. The influence of population size increased by 34 per cent; the influence of crop production per capita (affluence) increased by 11 per cent; the influence of the change in fertilizer technology increased by 405 per cent. Clearly the last factor dominates the large increase in the total environmental impact of fertilizer nitrogen. Specifically, it should be noted that in 1949 about 11,000 tons of fertilizer nitrogen were used *per unit crop production*, while in 1968 about 57,000 tons of nitrogen were employed for the *same* crop yield. This means that the efficiency with which fertilizer nitrogen contributes to crop yield has *declined* five fold. Obviously an appreciable part of the added nitrogen does not enter the crop and must appear elsewhere in the ecosystem.

The biological basis for this effect can be seen by comparing the corn yield in the State of Illinois, with the concurrent amounts of nitrogen fertilizer added to the soil. This shows that as fertilizer levels increased, the yield per acre rose, but eventually leveled off due to the natural limits of plant growth. Thus, between 1962 and 1968, fertilizer usage doubled, but crop yield rose only about 10 to 15 per cent. Clearly at the higher levels of fertilizer usage an increasingly small proportion of the fertilizer contributes to the crop. As indicated earlier, the remainder leaches into surface waters where it causes serious pollution problems. Thus, this innovation in agricultural technology sharply increases the environmental stress due to agricultural production.

A similar situation exists in the case of pesticides. This is shown by the changes in the environmental impact index of pesticides between 1950 and 1967 (Table 3). In that time there was a 168 per cent increase in the amount of pesticides used *per unit crop production*, as a national average. By killing off natural insect predators and parasites of the target pest, while the latter often becomes resistant to insecticides, the use of modern synthetic insecticides tends to exacerbate the pest problems that they were designed to control. As a result *increasing* amounts of insecticides must be used to maintain agricultural productivity. Insecticide usage is, so to speak, self-accelerating—resulting in both a decreased efficiency and an increased environmental impact.

Another technological displacement in agriculture is the increased use of feedlots for the production of livestock in preference to range feeding. Range-fed cattle are integrated into the soil ecosystem; they graze the soil's grass crop and restore nutrient to the soil as manure. When the cattle are maintained instead in huge pens, where they are fed on corn and deposit their wastes intensively in the feedlot itself, the wastes do not return to the soil. Instead the waste drains into

TABLE 3
Synthetic Organic Pesticides

	Index Factors			Total Index
	a	b	c	(a × b × c)
	Population (1000's)	Crop Production Population (Crop Production Units/cap.)	Pesticide Consumption Crop Production (1000 lb./Prod. Unit)	Synthetic Organic Pesticides (Million lb.)
1950	151,868	5.66×10^{-7}	3326	286
1967	197,859	5.96×10^{-7}	8898	1050
1967:1950	1.30	1.05	2.68	3.67
Increase, %	30	5	168	267

surface waters where it adds to the stresses due to fertilizer nitrogen and detergent phosphate. The magnitude of the effect is considerable. At the present time the organic waste produced in feedlots is more than the organic waste produced by all the cities of the United States. Again, the newer technology has a serious environmental impact, and in this case has displaced a technology with an essentially zero environmental impact.

Textiles

While total fiber production per capita has remained constant since 1946, natural fibers (cotton and wool) have been significantly displaced by synthetic ones. This technological change considerably increases the environmental impact due to fiber production and use.

One reason is that the energy required for the synthesis of the final product, a linear polymer (cellulose in the case of cotton, keratin in the case of wool, and polyamides in the case of nylon) is greater for the snythetic material. Although quantitative data are not yet available, this is evident from the comparison of two productive processes provided by Table 4. Nylon production involves as many as ten steps of chemical synthesis, each requiring considerable energy in the form of heat and electric power to overcome the entropy associated with chemical mixtures and to operate the reaction apparatus. In contrast, energy required for the synthesis of cotton is derived, free, from a renewable source—sunlight—and is transferred without combustion and resultant air pollution. Moreover, the raw material for cellulose synthesis is carbon dioxide and water, both freely available renewable resources, while the raw material for nylon synthesis is petroleum or a similar hydrocarbon—nonrenewable resources. As a result it would appear that the environmental stress due to the production of such an artificial fiber is probably well in excess of that due to the production of an equal weight of cotton. This is only an approximation, for we need far more detailed, quantitative estimates, in the form of the appropriate environmental impact indices, that would also take into account the fuel and other materials used in the production of cotton.

TABLE 4
Cotton and Nylon: Environmental Characteristics

	Cotton	*Nylon*	*Comparative Environmental Impact*
Raw Materials	CO_2, H_2O	Petroleum	Cotton, renewable Nylon, nonrenewable
Process	$CO_2 + H_2O$ light → glucose → cellulose (ca 70-90°F.) cultivation, ginning, spinning, require power	Petroleum (distill) → Benzene (550°F.) → Cyclohexane (300°F.) → Cyclohexanol (200-400°F.)→ Adipic acid (600-700°F.) → Adiponitrile (200-250°F.) → Hexamethylene diamine → Nylon 610 Disstillation and other purification at most of above steps; power required to operate process	Fuel combustion and resultant air pollution: probably Nylon greater than Cotton
Product	Cellulose	Polyamide	Cellulose wholly biodegradable, Polyamide not degradable

Because a synthetic fiber such as nylon is unnatural, it also has a greater impact on the environment as a waste material, than do cotton or wool. The natural polymers in cotton and wool, cellulose and keratin, are important constituents of the soil ecosystem. Through the action of molds and decay bacteria they contribute to the formation of humus. In this process cellulose is readily broken down in the soil ecosystem. Thus, in nature, cellulose and keratin are simply not wastes, because they provide essential nutrients for soil microorganisms. Hence they cannot accumulate. This results from the crucial fact that for every polymer which is produced in nature by living things, there exist in some living things enzymes which have the specific capability of degrading that polymer. In the absence of such an enzyme the natural polymers are quite resistant to degradation, as is evident from the durability of fabrics which are protected from biological attack.

The contrast with synthetic fibers is striking. The structure of nylon and similar synthetic polymers is a human invention and does not occur in natural living things. Hence, unlike natural polymers, synthetic ones find no counterpart in the armamentarium of degradative enzymes in nature. Ecologically, synthetic polymers are literally indestructible. Hence, every bit of synthetic fiber or polymer that has been produced on the earth is either destroyed by burning—and thereby pollutes the air—or accumulates as rubbish. One result, according to a recent report, is that microscopic fragments of plastic fibers, often red, blue, or orange, have now become common in certain marine waters. For technological displacement has been at work in this area too. In recent years natural fibers such as hemp and jute have been nearly totally replaced by synthetic fibers in fishing operations. A chief reason for this use of synthetic fibers is that they resist degradation by molds, which, as already indicated, readily attack cellulosic net materials such as hemp or jute. Thus, the property which enhances the economic value of the synthetic fiber over the natural one—its resistance to biological degradation—is precisely the property which increases the environmental impact of the synthetic material.

Detergents

Since 1946 synthetic detergents have largely replaced soap in the United States as domestic and industrial cleaners, with the total production of cleaners per capita remaining essentially unchanged. Soap is based on a natural organic substance, fat, which is reacted with alkali to produce the end product. Being a natural product, fat is extracted from an ecosystem (for example that represented by a coconut palm plantation), and when released into an aquatic ecosystem after use, soap is readily degraded by the bacteria of decay. Since most municipal wastes in the United States are subjected to treatment which degrades organic waste to its inorganic products, in actual practice the fatty residue of soap wastes is degraded by bacterial action within the confines of a sewage treatment plant. What is then emitted to surface waters is only carbon dioxide and water. Hence, there is little or no impact on the aquatic ecosystem due to biological oxygen demand (which accompanies bacterial degradation of organic wastes) arising from soap wastes. Nor is the product of soap degradation, carbon dioxide, usually an important ecological intrusion since it is in plentiful supply from other environmental sources, and in any case is an essential nutrient for photosynthetic algae.

Compared with soap the production of synthetic detergents is a more serious source of pollution. Once used and released into the environment in waste, detergents generate a more intense environmental impact than a comparable amount of soap. Soap is wholly degradable to carbon dioxide, which is usually rather innocuous in the environment. In contrast even the newer detergents, regarded as degradable because the paraffin chain of the molecule (being unbranched, in contrast with the earlier nondegradable detergents) is broken down by bacterial action, nevertheless leave a residue of phenol which may not be degraded and may accumulate in surface waters. Phenol is a rather toxic substance, being foreign to the aquatic ecosystem.

Unlike soap, detergents are compounded with considerable amounts of phosphate in order to enhance their cleansing action and as a water softener. Phosphate may readily induce water pollution by stimulating heavy overgrowths of algae, which on dying release organic matter into the water and thus overburden the aqueous ecosystem. Figure 3 shows that nearly all of the increase in sewage phosphorus in the United States can be accounted for by the phosphorus content of detergents. Since soap, which has been displaced by detergents, is quite free of phosphate the environmental impact due to phosphate is clearly a consequence of the technological change in cleaner production.

The change in the environmental impact index of phosphate in cleaners between 1946 and 1968 is shown in Table 5. In this period the overall environmental impact index increased 1845 per cent. The increase in the effect of population size was 42 per cent; the effect of per capita use of cleaners does not change; the technological factor, that due to the displacement of phosphate-free soap by detergents containing an average of about 4 per cent phosphorus, increased about 1270 per cent. The relative importance of this change in cleaner technology in intensifying environmental impact is quite evident.

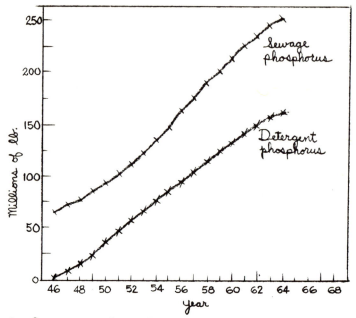

Figure 3: Concurrent values of phosphorus output from municipal sewage in the United States and phosphorus content of detergents produced. Sewage values are from Weinberger, L.W., et al. in Hearings before the Subcommittee on Science, Research, and Development, The Adequacy of Technology for Pollution Abatement, Vol. II, U. S. Government Printing Office, Washington, D. C., p. 756.

Secondary environmental effects of technological displacements

Increased production of synthetic organic chemicals leads to intensified environmental impacts in several different ways. This segment of industry has heavy power requirements; in contributing to increased power production the industry adds as well to the rising levels of air pollutants that are emitted by power plants. In addition, organic synthesis releases into the environment a wide variety of reagents and intermediates. These are foreign to natural ecosystems and are often toxic, thus generating important, often poorly understood, environmental impacts. Common examples are massive fish kills and plant damage resulting from release of organic wastes, insecticides, and herbicides to surface waters or the air.

Perhaps the most serious environmental impact attributable to the increased production of synthetic organic chemicals is due to the intrusion of mercury into surface waters. This effect is mediated by chlorine production. Chlorine is a vital reagent in many organic syntheses; about 80 per cent of present chlorine production finds its end

TABLE 5
Detergent Phosphorus, Environmental Impact Index

	Index Factors			*Total Impact*
	a	*b*	*c*	*(a × b × c)*
	Population	*Cleaners*[1] *Population*	*Phosphorus Cleaners*	*Phosphorus from Detergents*[2]
	(1000's)	*(lb./cap)*	*(lb./ton of cleaner)*	*(10^6 lb.)*
1946	140,686	22.66	6.90	11
1968	194,846	15.99	137.34	214
1968:1946	1.42	0.69 (1.00)[3]	19.90 (13.70)	19.45
Increase, % 1946-1968	42	(0)	(1,270)	1,845

[1]Assuming that 35% of detergent weight is active agent.

[2]Assuming average phosphorus content of detergents = 4%.

[3]Because of uncertainties regarding the content of active agent in detergents, especially soon after their introduction, the apparent reduction in per capita use of cleaners is not regarded as significant; the numbers contained in parentheses are based on the assumption that this value does not change significantly.

use in the synthetic organic chemical industry. Moreover, a considerable proportion of chlorine production is carried out in electrolytic mercury cells. Until recent control measures were imposed on the industry, about .2 to .5 lb. of mercury were released to the environment per ton of chlorine manufactured in mercury electrolytic cells. This means, for example, that the substitution of nylon for cotton has generated an intensified environmental impact due to mercury, for nylon production (unlike cotton production) involves the use of chlorinated intermediates, therefore of chlorine, and hence the release of mercury into the environment. The rapid, parallel rise in production of synthetic organic chemicals and chlorine production, and of the use of mercury for the latter is illustrated in Figure 4.

Similarly, the displacement of steel and lumber by aluminum adds to the burden of air pollutants, for aluminum production is extremely power consumptive. Per pound of aluminum produced, about 29,860 BTU's of power are required to generate the necessary electricity whereas about 4,615 BTU's are used per pound of steel produced. Cement, which tends to displace steel in construction, is also extremely power consumptive. The production of chemicals, aluminum,

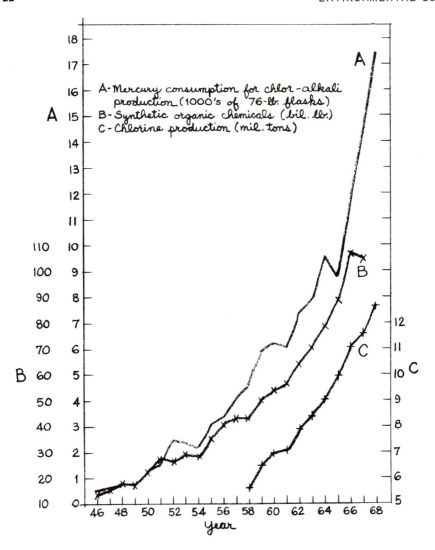

Figure 4: Changes in annual production of synthetic organic compounds and of chlorine gas, and consumption of mercury for chlorine gas production in the United States since 1946. Data are from Bureau of the Census, Current Industrial Reports, Series M28A Inorganic Chemicals and Gases and from Statistical Abstract of the United States, op cit.

and cement account for about 28 per cent of the total industrial use of electricity in the United States.

Packaging

The displacement of older forms of packaging by "disposable" containers, such as nonreturnable bottles, is another example of the intensification of environmental impact due to the postwar pattern of U.S. economic growth. This is illustrated in Figure 5 and Table 6. Here it is evident that there has been a very striking increase in environmental impact due to beer bottles, which are not assimilated by ecological systems and are, in their manufacture, quite power consumptive. It is also evident that the major factor in this intensified environmental impact is the new technology—the use of nonreturnable bottles to contain beer—rather than affluence with respect to per capita consumption of beer, or increased population. At the same time a recent study shows that the total expenditure of energy (for bottle manufacture, processing, shipping, etc.) required to deliver equal amounts of fluid in nonreturnable bottles is 4.7 times that for returnable ones.

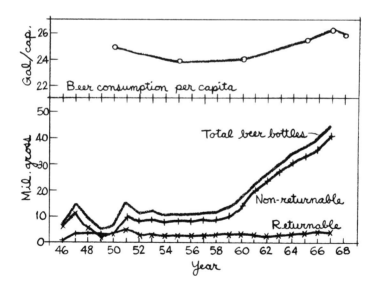

Figure 5: Per capita consumption of beer and production of beer bottles in the United States. Data are from Statistical Abstract of the United States, op cit., 1951, p. 792; 1955, p. 833; 1970, p. 12.

TABLE 6
Beer Bottles, Environmental Impact Index

	Index Factors			Total Index
	a	b	c	(a × b × c)
	Population (1000's)	Beer Consumption / Population (Gallons/cap)	Beer Bottles / Beer Consumption (Bottles/gallon)	Beer Bottles (1000 Gross)
1950	151,868	24.99	.25	6,540
1967	197,859	26.27	1.26	45,476
1967:1950	1.30	1.05	5.08	6.95
Increase, % 1950-1967	30	5	408	595

Automotive Vehicles

Finally there is the problem of assessing the environmental impact of changes in patterns of passenger travel and freight traffic since 1946. Particularly important has been the increased use of automobiles, busses and trucks.

The environmental impact of the internal combustion engine is due to the emission of nitrogen oxides, carbon monoxide, waste fuel, and lead. The intensities of these impacts, as measured by the levels of these pollutants in the environment is a function, not only of the vehicle-miles travelled, but also of the nature of the engine itself-technological factors are relevant as well.

The technological changes in automotive engines since World War II have worsened environmental impact. These are illustrated in Figure 6. Thus, for passenger automobiles, overall mileage per gallon of fuel declined from 14.97 in 1949 to 14.08 in 1967, largely because average horsepower increased from 100 to 240. Another important technological change was in average compression ratio, which increased from about 5.9 to 9.5 in 1946-68. This engineering change has had two important effects on the environmental impact of the gasoline engine. First increasing amounts of tetraethyl lead are needed as a gasoline additive in order to suppress the engine knock that occurs at high compression ratios. Annual use of tetraethyl lead has increased more than fivefold between 1946 and 1968. Essentially all of this lead is emitted from the engine exhaust and is disseminated into the environment. Since

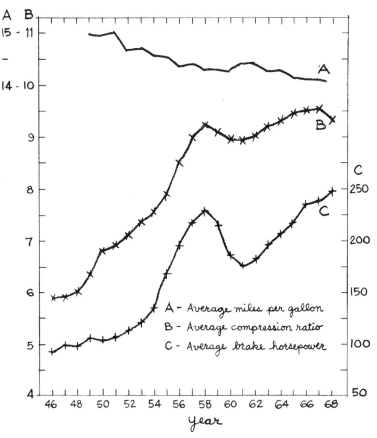

Figure 6: Average characteristics of passenger car engines produced in the United States since 1946. Brake horsepower and compression ratio data are from the 1951 and 1970 volumes of "Brief Passenger Car Data," Ethyl Corporation. Gasoline consumption data are from Statistical Abstract of the United States, op cit.

lead is not a functional element in any biological organism, and is in fact toxic, it represents an external intrusion on the ecosystem and generates an appreciable environmental effect.

A second consequence of the increase in engine compression ratio has been a rise in the concentration of nitrogen oxides emitted in engine exhaust. This has occurred because the engine temperature increases with compression ratio. The combination of nitrogen and oxygen, present in the air taken into the engine cylinder, to form nitrogen oxides is enhanced at elevated temperatures. Nitrogen oxide is the key ingredient in the formation of photochemical smog. Through a series of light-activated reactions, involving waste fuel, nitrogen oxides induce the formation of peroxyacetyl nitrate, the noxious ingredient

of photochemical smog. Smog of this type was first detected in Los
Angeles in 1942; it was unknown in most other United States cities
until the late 1950's and 1960's, but is now a nearly universal urban
pollutant. Peroxyacetyl nitrate is a toxic agent, to man, agricultural
crops, and trees. Introduction of this agent has probably increased by
about an order of magnitude in the period 1946 to 1968.

The Environmental Impact Indices for nitrogen oxides and lead are
shown in Tables 7 and 8 respectively. The total environmental impact
for nitrogen oxides increased by about 630 per cent between 1946 and
1967. The technological factor (the amount of nitrogen oxides emitted
per vehicle mile) increased by 158 per cent, vehicle miles travelled
per capita increased by about 100 per cent, and the population factor
by about 41 per cent. In the case of tetraethyl lead, the largest increase in impact is in vehicle miles travelled per capita (100%), followed by the technological factor (83%) and the population factor (41%).
It is evident that the major influences on automotive air pollution are
increased per capita mileage (in part because of changes in work-
residence distribution caused by expansion of suburbs) and the increased environmental impact per mile travelled caused by technological changes in the gasoline engine.

TABLE 7
Nitrogen Oxides (Passenger Vehicles)
Environmental Impact Index

	Index Factors			Total Index
	a	b	c	$(a \times b \times c)$
	Population (1000's)	Vehicle-Miles Population	Nitrogen Oxides[1] Vehicle-miles	Nitrogen Oxides[1]
1946	140,686	1982	33.5	10.6
1967	197,849	3962	86.4	77.5
1967:1946	1.41	2.00	2.58	7.3
Increase, %	41	100	158	630

[1]Dimension = NOx (ppm) × gasoline consumption (gals. × 10^{-6}). Estimated from
product of passenger vehicle gasoline consumption and ppm of NOx emitted by engines
of average compression ratio 5.9 (1946) and 9.5 (1967) under running conditions, at
15 in. manifold pressure: 1946, 500 ppm NOx; 1967, 1200 ppm.

TABLE 8
Tetraethyl Lead, Environmental Impact Index

	Index Factors			*Total Index*
	a	*b*	*c*	
	Population *(1000's)*	*Vehicle-Miles*[1] *Population* *(vehicle mi./cap)*	*Tetraethyl Lead*[2] *Vehicle-miles*[1] *(lb./million vehicle mi.)*	*Tetraethyl Lead*[2] *(1000's of tons)*
1946	140,686	1984[3]	300[3]	48[3]
1967	197,859	3962	630	247
1967:1946	1.41	2.00	1.83	5.15
Increase, %	41	100	83	415

[1]Passenger vehicles only.
[2]Weight refers to lead content.
[3]See note for Table IX.

A similar situation obtains with respect to overland shipments of intercity freight. Here truck freight has tended to displace railroad freight. And again the displacing technology has a more severe environmental impact than does the displaced technology. This is evident from the energy required to transport freight by rail and truck: 624 BTU/ton-mile by rail and 3462 BTU/ton-mile by truck. It should be noted as well that the steel and cement required to produce equal lengths of railroad and expressway (suitable for heavy truck traffic) differ in the amount of power required in the ratio 1 to 3.6. This is due to the rather power-consumptive nature of cement production and to the fact that four highway lanes are required to accommodate heavy truck traffic. In addition, the divided roadway requires a 400 foot right-of-way while a train roadbed needs only 100 feet. In all these ways the displacement of railroads by automotive vehicles, not only for freight, but also for passenger travel, has intensified the resultant environmental impact.

THE ENVIRONMENTAL IMPACT INVENTORY

It will be recognized that the foregoing analysis represents only small fragments of a complex whole. What is required is a full inventory of the various Environmental Impact Indices associated with the productive enterprise and the identification of the origins of these impacts within the production process and of the ecosystems on which they intrude. Such an assemblage of data, representing an Environmental Impact Inventory is derived as an exploratory exercise in what follows, with reference to a productive item for which a certain amount of the needed data happen to be at hand—the production of chlorine and alkali by chloralkali plants employing mercury electrolytic cells.

The needed data include: (a) The Environmental Impact Indices associated with the input goods, chiefly, electric power, salt, and mercury; (b) The Environmental Impact Indices representative of the process's wastes and the properties of the ecological systems which are affected by them; (c) The Environmental Impact Indices representative of the ecologically significant wastes associated with the process' output goods (chlorine and alkali) and the environmental fate of this material. Thus, the production of 1 megawatt of electricity by fossil-fuel burning plants results in the release of 34.20 lb. of sulfur oxides to the atmosphere. Since 4300 kwh is consumed by a mercury cell chloralkali plant, per ton of chlorine produced, on the average, 147 lbs. of sulfur oxides are released to the environment per ton of chlorine produced. In this way the corresponding values for other power-plant pollutants (nitrogen oxides, dust) can be computed as well.

The major ecologically significant waste from chloralkali production is mercury metal. Two studies provide data on the amounts of mercury released to the air, to surface waters, or buried in land-fill, per ton of chlorine produced. For example, per ton of chlorine produced, about 17 to 35 gm. of mercury vapor is emitted to the air as waste. Chemical engineering data indicate a total "mercury loss" of .2 to .5 lb. per ton of chlorine for the process. This agrees rather well with the total losses to the environment estimated directly by the foregoing studies, .13 to .57 lb. of mercury per ton of chlorine.

The present data indicate that as much as 20 grams of mercury may become incorporated in the alkali produced in the course of producing a ton of chlorine; this alkali is used in some 42 separate products. From an input-output analysis of the chloralkali industry one could construct a comprehensive matrix for the movement of mercury contained in alkali through various manufacturing processes into the environment. Recently, economic input-output methods have been adapted to include environmental externalities. For the present purposes we shall restrict the analysis to a group of products—wood pulp and paper, soap, lye, and cleansers—which use about 26 per cent of the alkali output. Hence, we may estimate that of every 20 grams of mercury which goes into alkali, 26 per cent, or 5 grams, appears in the products listed above.

The environmental fates of these products are known: waste water containing cleansers goes into waterways, as do the fluid wastes from pulp and paper production; paper is eventually burned, releasing its mercury to the air as vapor.

The ecological data relevant to an Environmental Impact Inventory for chloralkali production are just beginning to be investigated. When metallic mercury is dumped into surface waters it sinks into the bottom mud, as droplets. There it may be acted on by certain species of bacteria which convert the mercury to an organic form, methyl mercury. While metallic mercury does not dissolve in water, methyl mercury does. Hence in this form the mercury is readily taken up by living organisms in the water, ultimately contaminating fish that may be eaten by people. In recent months it has been found that mercury wastes from a number of chloralkali plants have caused mercury levels in fish in adjacent surface water to exceed acceptable public health limits. Emitted into the air, mercury may be taken up directly by human beings through absorption in the lungs, or may be washed down into soil and water by precipitation—and thus enter these ecosystems. Very little is known about the ecological transfer of mercury in the soil. Finally, since mercury is very volatile, when heated (as in an incinerator) it is vaporized and emitted into the air. A recent study shows that St. Louis domestic incinerators emit about 2,000 to 3,000 lb. of mercury into the air annually. Much of this originates in the incineration of paper and wood pulp products.

On the basis of such data one can now produce (here in a quite incomplete and tentative form) an Environmental Impact Inventory for chloralkali production. This is presented in Table 9.

SOME CONCLUSIONS

The data presented above reveal a functional connection between economic growth—at least in the United States since 1946—and environmental impact. It is significant that the range of increase in the computed environmental impacts agrees fairly well with the independent measure of the actual levels of pollutants occurring in the environment. Thus, the increase in environmental impact index for tetraethyl lead computed from gasoline consumption data for 1946 to 1968 is about 400 per cent; a similar increase in environmental lead levels has been recorded from analyses of layered ice in glaciers. Similarly, the 648 per cent increase in the 19-year period 1949-1968 in the environmental impact index computed for nitrogen fertilizer is in keeping with the few available large-scale field measurements. Thus, field data show that

TABLE 9
Environmental Impact Inventory
Chloralkali production by means of mercury electrolytic cells

	Production Process	Relevant Ecological Systems[2]	Environmental Impact (per ton of chlorine produced)
Input Goods[1]	Electric Power (4300 kwh/ton Cl)	Air	SO_x: 147.1 lb. NO_x: 29.4 lb. Particulates: 5.9 lb. Mercury: .004 gm. Heat: 5.51×10^6 Btu's
		Surface waters	Heat: 16.56×10^6 Btu's
	H_2 gas ventilation	Air	Mercury: 17-35 gm.
Production Process Step[1]	H_2 condensate, wash water	Surface waters via settling pond or drainage system	Mercury: 35-121 gm.
	Brine sludge removal	Surface waters	
	Anode Sweepings removal	Soil via land fill	Mercury: 6-97 gm.
Output Goods[1]	Selected alkali-using goods (soap, lye, cleansers, pulp and paper)	Air Surface waters	Mercury: 1-5 gm.

Total Mercury: 59-258gm./ton chlorine (.10-.57 lb./ton chlorine)

[1] Only a few of the actual items are shown, for purposes of illustration.
[2] In an actual index reference would be made to a standardized desctiption of each of the indicated relevant ecological systems.

nitrate entering the Missouri River as it traversed Nebraska in the 6-year period 1956 to 1962 increased a little over 200 per cent. The environmental impact indices computed for several aspects of automotive vehicle use are also in keeping with general field observations. It is widely recognized that the most striking increase among the several aspects of environmental deterioration due to automotive vehicles has occurred with respect to photochemical smog. Since its first detection in 1942, photochemical smog has increased, nationally, by probably an order of magnitude, appearing in nearly every major city and even in smaller ones in the last five years. However, in the period 1946 to 1968 total use of automotive vehicles, as measured by gasoline consumption, increased by only about 200 per cent—an increment too small to account for the concurrent rise in the incidence of photochemical smog. It is significant, then, that this disparity between the observed increase in smog levels and the increase in vehicle use is accounted for by the environmental impact index computed for nitrogen oxides, the agent which initiates the smog reaction, for that index increased by 630 per cent during the period 1946 to 1967.

These agreements with actual field data support the conclusion that the computations represented by the environmental impact index provide a useful approximation of the changes in environmental impact associated with the relevant features of the growth of the United States economy since 1946. In particular, we can therefore place some reliance on the subdivision of the total impact index into the several factors: population size, per capita production or consumption and the technology of production and use.

It is interesting to make a direct comparison of the relative contributions of increases in population size and in affluence, and of changes in the technology of production, to the increases in total environmental impact which have occurred since 1946. The ratio of the most recent total index value to the value of the 1946 index (or to the value for the earliest year for which the necessary data are available) is indicative of the change in the total impact over this period of time. The relative contributions of the several factors to these total changes are then given by the ratios of the logarithms of their respective partial indices. Figure 7 reports such comparisons for the six productive activities evaluated. The logarithm of the population factor contributes only between 12 and 20 per cent of the logarithm of the total change in impact index. For all but the automotive pollutants, the affluence factor expressed as a logarithm makes a rather small contribution— no more than 5 per cent—to the total changes in impact index. For nitrogen oxides and tetraethyl lead (from automotive sources), this factor accounts for about 40 per cent of the total effect, reflecting a

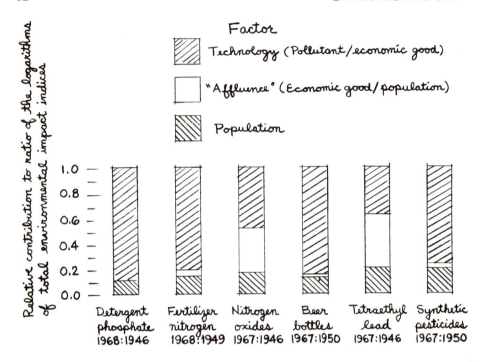

Figure 7: *Relative contributions of several factors to changes in environmental impact indices. The contributions of population size, "affluence" (production per capita), and technological characteristics (amount of pollutant released per unit production) to the total environmental impact indices were computed as shown in the text. Each bar is subdivided to show the relative contributions, on a scale of 1.0, of the several factors to the ratio of the total impact index value for the earlier year.*

considerable increase in the number of vehicle miles travelled per capita since 1946. The logarithm of the technological changes in the processes which generate the various economic goods, contribute from 40 to 90 per cent of the logarithm of the total increases in impact.

In evaluating these results it should be noted that automotive travel is itself strongly affected by a kind of technological transformation—the rapid increase of suburban residences in the United States and the concomitant failure to provide adequate railroad and other mass transportation to accommodate to this change. That the overall increase in vehicle miles travelled per capita since 1946 (about 100 per cent) is related to increased residence-work travel incident upon this change is suggested by the results of a 1963 survey. It was found that 90 per cent of all automobile trips, representing 30 per cent of total mileage travelled, are 10 miles or less in length. The mean residence-work travel distance was about 5.5 miles. Thus, it is probably appropriate to regard the increase in per capita vehicle miles travelled by automobile as not totally attributable to increased affluence, but rather as a response to new work-residence relationships which are costly in transportation.

During the period from 1946 to the present, pollution levels in the United States have increased sharply—generally by an order of magnitude or so. It seems evident from the data presented above that most of this increase is due to one of the three factors that influence environmental impact—the technology of production—and that both population growth and increase in affluence exert a much smaller influence. Thus the chief reason for the sharp increase in environmental stress in the United States is the sweeping transformation in production technology in the postwar period. Productive activities with intense environmental impacts have displaced activities with less serious environmental impacts; the growth pattern has been counterecological.

The foregoing conclusion is easily misconstrued to mean that technology is therefore, *per se*, ecologically harmful. That this interpretation is unwarranted can be seen from the following examples.

Consider the following simple transformation of the present, ecologically faulty, relationship among soil, agricultural crops, the human population, and sewage. Suppose that the sewage, instead of being introduced into surface waters as it is now, whether directly or following treatment, is instead transported from urban collection systems by pipeline to agricultural areas, where—after appropriate sterilization procedures—it is incorporated into the soil. Such a pipeline would literally reincorporate the urban population into the soil's ecological cycle, restoring the integrity of that cycle, and incidentally removing the need for inorganic nitrogen fertilizer—which also stresses the aquatic cycle. Hence the urban population is then no longer external to the soil cycle and is therefore incapable either of generating a negative biological stress upon it or of exerting a positive ecological stress on the aquatic ecosystem. But note that this state of zero environmental impact is not achieved by a return to primitive conditions, but by an actual technological advance, the construction of a sewage pipeline system.

Or consider the example provided by the technological treatment of gold and other precious metals. Gold is, after all, subject to numerous technological manipulations, which generate a series of considerable economic values. Yet we manage to accomplish all of this without intruding more than a rather small fraction of all the gold ever acquired by human beings into the ecosphere. Because we value it so highly very little gold is lost to the environment. In contrast, most of the mercury which has entered commerce in the last generation has been disseminated into the environment, with very unfortunate effects on the environment. Clearly, given adequate technology—and motivation—we could be as thrifty in our handling of mercury as we are of gold, thereby preventing the entry of this toxic material into the environment. Again what is required is not necessarily the abandonment of mercury-based technology, but rather the improvement of that technology to the point of satisfactory compatability with the ecosystem.

Generally speaking then, it would appear possible to reduce the environmental impact of human activities by developing alternatives to ecologically faulty activities. This can be accomplished, not by abandoning technology and the economic goods which it can yield, but by developing new technologies which incorporate not only the knowledge of the physical sciences (as most do moderately well; the new machines do, after all, usually produce their intended goods), but ecological wisdom as well.

We come, then, to the matter of the actual cost of the degradation which has been the response of the environmental system to the intensified impacts upon it. This is, of course, a very difficult matter. As indicated earlier the theory which links environmental impact to ecological effect is for the most part poorly developed. At the same time there are formidable difficulties confronting the economist who attempts to return the externalities represented by ecological damage to the realm of economic evaluation. These efforts, which appear to be developing increasingly useful information, need not be reviewed here. For there is, I believe, a simpler and more direct way to express the cost to the economic system represented by environmental deterioration.

It seems to me that a meaningful way to evaluate this cost is somewhat along the following lines:

1. Given that the deterioration of the environment, whatever its cost in money, social distress, and personal suffering, is, as shown in the foregoing analysis, chiefly the result of the ecologically faulty technology which has been employed to remake productive enterprises in the United States since 1946;

2. And given that the resulting environmental impacts stress the basic ecosystems which support the life of human beings, destroy the biological capital which is essential to the operation of industry and agriculture, and may in a period of a few decades lead to the catastrophic collapse of these systems;

3. And given further that the environmental impacts already generated are sufficient to threaten the continued development of the economic system—witness the difficulties in siting new power plants at

a time of severe power shortage, the recent curtailment of industrial innovation in the fields of detergents, chemical manufacturing, pesticides, herbicides, chlorine production, oil drilling, oil transport, supersonic aviation, nuclear power generation, industrial uses of nuclear explosives, all resulting from public rejection of the concomitant environmental deterioration;

4. Then it seems probably, if we are to survive economically as well as biologically, that much of the technological transformation of the United States economy since 1946 will need to be, so to speak, redone in order to bring the nation's productive technology much more closely into harmony with the inescapable demands of the ecosystem. This will require the development of massive new technologies including: systems to return sewage and garbage directly to the soil; for the replacement of synthetic materials by natural ones; to support the reversal of the present trend to retire soil from agriculture and to elevate the yield per acre; for the development of land transport that operates with maximal fuel efficiency at low combustion temperatures; to enable the sharp curtailment of the use of biologically active synthetic organic agents. In effect what is required is a new period of technological transformation of the economy, which reverses the counterecological trends developed since 1946. We might estimate the cost of the new transformation, from the cost of the former one, which must represent a capital investment in the range of hundreds of billions of dollars. To this must be added, of course, the cost of repairing the ecological damage which has already been incurred, such as the eutrophication of Lake Erie, again a bill to be reckoned in the hundreds of billions of dollars.

The enormous size of these costs raises a final question. Is there some functional connection in the economy between the tendency of a given productive activity to inflict an intense impact on the environment (and the size of the resultant costs) and the role of this activity in economic growth? For it is evident from even a cursory comparison of the productive activities which have rapidly expanded in the United States economy since 1946 with the activities which they have displaced, that the displacing activities are also considerably more profitable than those which they displace. The correlation between profitability and rapid growth is one that is presumably accountable by economics. Is the additional linkage to intense environmental impact also functional, or only accidental?

It has been pointed out often enough that environmental pollution represents a long-unpaid debt to nature. Is it possible that the United States economy has grown since 1946 by deriving much of its new wealth through the enlargement of that debt? If this should turn out to be the case what strains will develop in the economy if, for the sake of the survival of our society, that debt should now be called? How will these strains affect our ability to pay the debt—to survive?

SUGGESTED READING

Weinberger, L. W., Stephan, D. G., and Middleton, F. M., *Annals New York Academy of Sciences*, 136:131, 1966.

Commoner, B., Threats to the Integrity of the Nitrogen Cycle: Nitrogen Compounds in Soil, Water, Atmosphere and Precipitation, *in* Singer, S. F., *ed., Global Effects of Environmental Pollution*, Symposium organized by American Association for the Advancement of Science, Dallas, Texas, December 1968, Reidel, Dordrecht-Holland 1970.

PEOPLE WHO LIVE IN GAS HOUSES

The Greenhouse Effect, Man's Influence on Climate

Theodore L. Brown

Earth is blanketed by an ocean of gas which we call the atmosphere. Without the protective cover of the atmosphere life as we know it would be impossible. Aside from the obvious ways in which the atmosphere enables life forms to exist, it plays many vital roles in determining climate. The massive alterations of the atmosphere that man is producing may affect climate on a global scale and in turn, may change the kind of life that can thrive.

We can identify three major ways in which man's energy-generating activity affects the global climate. In the first place, he adds infrared absorbers to the earth's atmosphere. Secondly, his activities generate particulate matter, finely divided solid material dispersed in the atmosphere and remaining there for a long time. There dispersions are aerosols. Thirdly, man may affect the global climate by simply dissipating energy that competes with the incoming solar radiation.

THE INFRARED ABSORBERS

To understand the effect of adding infrared absorbing gases to the atmosphere, we must review a few things about electromagnetic radiation. The various forms of electromagnetic radiation with which we are familiar, including visible light, radio waves, x-rays, and infrared radiation, are similar in that they all move through space with the characteristic speed of light, and each has associated with it a characteristic wavelength. We talk about wavelength in units of microns. A micron is a millionth of a meter, and a meter is slightly longer than a yard. The visible radiation to which our eyes are sensitive lies in a region of the spectrum where the wavelength is about half a micron. Radiation at higher energy—and that means shorter wavelength—consists of the so-called ultraviolet rays. At longer wavelengths and lower energies is infrared radiation.

Although we may seldom be aware of the fact, every object radiates energy and has a temperature associated with it. For example, a lump of charcoal at room temperature looks black and is radiating energy of very long wavelength, as is characteristic of a relatively cool object. If the charcoal is heated, it eventually gets hot enough that it emits visible radiation. Heated to still higher temperature, it glows with a white heat; an extremely hot object radiates a blue light. The radiation which emanates from an object is therefore related to its temperature. Figure 1 shows two examples of black-body radiation, the radiation at a given temperature of a material which absorbs all incident radiation. The vertical axes in the graphs show levels of energy (calories/square centimeter/minute/unit wavelength). The horizontal axes are divided in units of wavelength.

Figure 1A depicts the black-body radiation curve, as it is called, for an object at 11,000°F (Fahrenheit) (6,000°C). This is approximately the temperature of the surface of the sun. In effect, Figure 1A shows the energy distribution of the radiation coming from the sun. Notice that the peak is at about 0.5 micron, in the middle of the visible range of the spectrum, and that this maximum corresponds to an energy output of about 15,000 calories per square centimeter per minute. By contrast, note the second curve (Figure 1B), which depicts the black body radiation for an object at 80°F, just above room temperature. The maximum occurs at ten microns, a much longer wavelength than that of the sun's radiation. Furthermore, the amount of energy per square centimeter per minute is very much smaller. The maximum is only about .045, whereas on the solar curve it is 15,000. If the 80°F blackbody radiation curve were plotted on the 11,000°F graph, the line would be indistinguishable from the base line.

The situation then is something like this: The sun radiates energy toward earth with the wavelength distribution shown in Figure 1A. The earth radiates energy into space distributed in wavelength according to curves closely similar to that in Figure 1B. Of course, the sun's radiation has a very, very high flux, or intensity, at the surface of the sun. But by the time it arrives at earth, 93 million miles away, the radiation has been spread out in space, so the amount per square

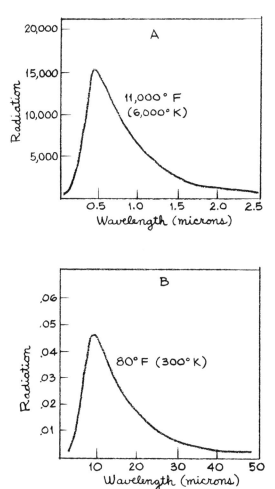

Figure 1: Black-body emission curves.

centimeter which reaches the surface of the earth is far smaller. To compare incoming and outgoing radiation, we must shrink the vertical scale in Figure 1A, without changing the wavelength maximum. The result is shown in Figure 2. The first curve shows the incoming solar radiation, still concentrated at 0.5 micron, but now very much reduced in intensity because of dissipation out into space. The second curve shows the black-body radiation from earth. Because the temperature of the earth in relatively stable, we know that the earth is, more or less, in balance with the solar radiation—the amount of energy coming in from the sun is equal to the amount of energy radiating from earth back into space. Recent data obtained from orbiting meteorological satellites confirm that the earth is indeed in approximate radiation balance.

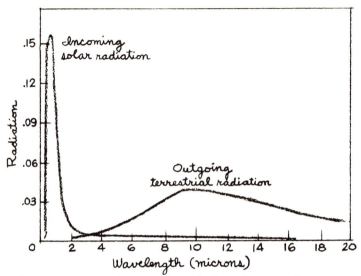

Figure 2: Comparison of the wavelength distributions for incoming solar radiation and outgoing radiation from the earth.

While the two curves of Figure 2 represent equal amounts of incoming and outgoing radiation, they show that the wavelengths of radiation involved differ dramatically. The wavelength maximum for incoming radiation is at 0.5 micron; the maximum for outgoing radiation is at about 10 microns. This fact, together with the presence of infrared absorbers in the atmosphere, have a major influence on climate.

Figure 3 shows the regions of the infrared spectrum in which the gases carbon dioxide, water, and ozone, are strongly absorbing. The figure also shows the black-body radiation curve for the earth (the same one shown in Figure 2) with a maximum at about ten microns. Ozone's effect is not significant; it has only one very narrow, intense, infrared absorption band. For our purposes, it is possible to ignore ozone altogether.

Water is the major absorber. It absorbs infrared radiation strongly, and is present in the atmosphere in great quantities. But notice that a third gas, carbon dioxide, does absorb rather strongly in a region where there is a "window" in the water absorption. This region is important because it comes very close to the maximum for the outgoing radiation from the earth. Thus radiation energy emitted by Earth is held by the infrared-absorbing gases H_2O and CO_2.

On the other hand, both water and carbon dioxide are transparent to visible light. They therefore do not significantly absorb light coming in from the sun. If they did, the atmosphere would look colored to us below it. To understand how CO_2 changes could affect climate we need to ask more questions. First, what about the distribution of H_2O and CO_2? Carbon dioxide is distributed in the atmosphere more or less uniformly at all altitudes. The so-called *mixing ratio* is about 315 parts per million. Water vapor, on the other hand, is very much differently distributed as a function of altitude. Near the surface of the earth there is a lot of water vapor in the atmosphere. On a warm, muggy day in Illinois there may be 20,000 parts per million of water vapor in the air. The water vapor level drops off very rapidly with increasing altitude until, at the boundary between the troposphere and stratosphere, 6 to 7 miles in altitude, the water mixing ratio is less than 10 parts per million. The concentrations of H_2O and CO_2 in the atmosphere are about equal at perhaps 4 miles altitude; above that, water vapor is much less prevalent than carbon dioxide.

Earth's surface has a certain temperature, and it radiates energy. The lowest layer of the atmosphere, containing substantial quantities of both water vapor and carbon dioxide, absorbs some of that radiation, but, because its temperature is not zero, it reradiates the energy it

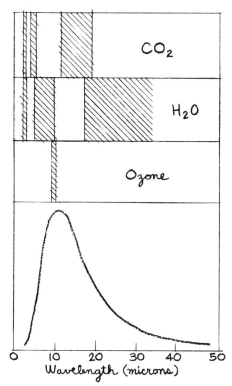

Figure 3: Absorption of infrared radiation by carbon dioxide, water, and ozone. The lower portion of the figure shows the wavelength distribution of the outgoing radiation from the earth.

absorbs. Part of the energy is radiated back towards the earth, and part upward into the next atmospheric layer. The next layer then receives the energy radiated from the first layer, and some fraction of the energy emitted by the surface. The second layer in turn radiates some energy up into the next higher layer and some back down. And as we go up from layer to layer, less and less energy from earth reaches those successive layers. The result is a decrease in temperature with increasing altitude. Figure 4 shows data on the temperature of the atmosphere as a function of altitude, obtained by an orbiting meteorological satellite over Green Bay, Wisconsin on April 11, 1969 at 11:00 P.M. The temperature of the atmosphere drops steadily with height to the top of the troposphere, near the layer called the *tropopause,* the interface between the troposphere and stratosphere. Above this, the temperature increases again, but this is not related to infrared absorption. The stratospheric temperature increase is related to what we might call the "ozone machine," resulting from a photochemical reaction of atmospheric oxygen, producing ozone. We are concerned, however, with the portion of the atmosphere within ten miles of the earth's surface.

The general temperature decrease with altitude in the troposphere is called the *lapse rate.* There are, of course, detailed differences in that curve from one place to another on the earth's surface and with the

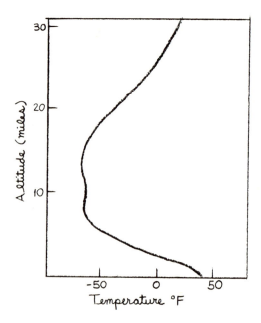

Figure 4: A typical profile of atmospheric temperature. The data for development of the temperature profile were obtained from a Nimbus III orbiting meteorological satellite.

time of day, and so on. In other words, although the atmospheric temperature profile reflects weather conditions which change from day to day, the general shape of the temperature profile remains the same.

The problem we have then is the following: What would happen if the amount of carbon dioxide in the atmosphere—now 315 parts per million were to increase greatly, say to double? How much change in the temperature at the surface of the earth and elsewhere in the temperature profile would occur as a result of an increase up to 600 parts per million? That is the kind of question we want to ask because that will be an indication of how important carbon dioxide might be in affecting the earth's climate. To answer the question we must have a model for the atmosphere, and the results of calculations based on the model, because we obviously can't do the experiment of doubling the carbon dioxide content in the atmosphere.

The design of a model for radiation effects on the atmosphere and the formulation of this model on a computer is complex. A number of attempts have been made. Some of the most recent work, done about five years ago at the Geophysical Fluid Dynamics Laboratory of the Environmental Sciences Service Administration in Washington, D. C., was carried out by Syukuro Manabe and Richard T. Wetherald. They constructed as realistic a model of the atmosphere as they could manage in terms of computer capability. It assumes a water vapor distribution in the atmosphere which matches experimental data, in that the water vapor pressure drops off markedly with increasing altitude, and the infrared absorption patterns for water and carbon dioxide shown in Figure 3. There are pressure effects that must be taken into account, so when one gets into the details, it is a very complicated calculation.

On the basis of their model, and assuming 300 parts per million of CO_2, Manabe and Wetherald calculated an atmospheric temperature profile that matched well the measured one shown in Figure 4. They then repeated the calculation assuming 600 parts per million of CO_2. They found that there is about 4°F higher temperature at the surface when the CO_2 level is doubled, assuming a constant relative humidity. Manabe and Wetherald's calculation tells us roughly what the effect of doubling the CO_2 level would be, but it suggests other questions. How much CO_2 is man putting into the atmosphere, and when is the level likely to double, if it ever does?

Table I shows the distribution of carbon dioxide. There are three places where relatively free carbon dioxide is to be found: in the atmosphere, dissolved in the oceans, and tied up in the biomass—in all the plant and animal matter on the earth. The amount of CO_2 in the atmosphere is 2.5 trillion (2.5×10^{12}) tons. The amount in the oceans is much larger—140 trillion tons. By comparison, the amount in the biomass, 1.5 trillion tons, is much smaller.

TABLE 1.

Distribution of CO_2 and Sources of Fossil Fuels.

Atmosphere	2.5×10^{12} tons CO_2
Oceans	140×10^{12} tons CO_2
Biomass	1.5×10^{12} tons CO_2
Coal	4.7×10^{12} tons C
Oil + Natural Gas	0.4×10^{12} tons C
Total Fuel	5.1×10^{12} tons C
	16×10^{12} tons CO_2

The second part of Table I lists data on the sources of fuels. These numbers are the estimated recoverable reserves of some of these fuels. If all these recoverable reserves of fossil fuels, which amount to about 5×10^{12} tons of carbon, were burned to form carbon dioxide, they would produce about 16×10^{12} tons of carbon dioxide, about six times greater the total quantity of carbon dioxide now in the atmosphere. There is, of course, an equilibrium involving exchange of carbon dioxide between the atmosphere and the oceans. We need to look into that balance to learn how much of the carbon dioxide put into the atmosphere is likely to remain there, how much will go into the oceans, and the time scale involved in the ocean-atmosphere interchange.

Exchange of atmospheric carbon dioxide with the ocean can be roughly divided into two stages. There is a fairly rapid exchange between the atmosphere and that two per cent of the total volume of the ocean which is the top layer. Turbulent, in continual turnover, the surface water is rapidly exposed to the atmosphere and exchanges carbon dioxide with the atmosphere rapidly. The half life for this rapid exchange process is on the order of a year or two. The other 98 per cent of the ocean is in very much slower equilibrium with atmospheric CO_2. Radiocarbon studies done on deep ocean water suggest that the half life for exchange of deep-water CO_2 with the atmosphere could be on the order of 1,000 to 4,000 years.

We can now do a simple exercise. If we assume that two per cent of the ocean is involved with the exchange, and if we assume that the carbon dioxide is more or less equally distributed throughout the oceans, as is in fact the case, we can go back to 140×10^{12} tons and take two per cent of that—2.8×10^{12} tons. Recall that there are about 2.5×10^{12} tons of CO_2 in the atmosphere. Therefore, if the atmospheric CO_2 content were to double, probably somewhat more than half the added CO_2 would dissolve in the ocean with a half life on the order of a year or two. Over a much longer period of time, from one thousand to four thousand years, much of the rest of the added CO_2 would dissolve in the oceans. These calculations provide a rough indication of how much added CO_2 might remain atmospheric. Luckily we need not depend upon these approximations because there are data which indicate what is happening to the carbon dioxide content of the atmosphere.

For a number of years Charles D. Keeling, Bert Bolin and their coworkers, have been measuring the carbon dioxide content of the atmosphere. Figure 5 shows the carbon dioxide content at Mauna Loa in Hawaii as a function of time during the period from late 1959 to early 1962. The atmosphere was sampled daily; the numbers shown are monthly averages of the carbon dioxide content. It is apparent that during this period the carbon dioxide content of the atmosphere, even in this locale supposedly quite free of pollution, was steadily increasing at a rate of about 0.7 part per million per year. To find out how the observed increase compares with the amount of carbon dioxide added by man during that period, we need estimates of world-wide fuel consumption. On the basis of United Nations data for 1960, which are included in the period of interest, we find about 4.6×10^9 tons of carbon equivalent in the form of fuel were used worldwide during that

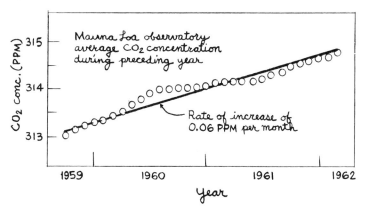

Figure 5: Annual average carbon dioxide concentrations, Mauna Loa, Hawaii.

year. That converts to 15×10^9 tons of carbon dioxide. Now, 0.7 part per million per year corresponds to addition of 5.5×10^9 tons of carbon dioxide being added to the atmosphere. We therefore reach the conclusion that during 1960 man presumably put into the atmosphere 15×10^9 tons of CO_2, and 5.5×10^9 tons stayed there. That corresponds to a retention of about forty per cent, not too far from our guess based on the very simpleminded considerations as described above. Since these two approaches seem to agree pretty well, we can assume as a working hypothesis that about 40 per cent of the CO_2 generated by man will remain in the atmosphere for a long time, the other 60 per cent presumably dissolving in the oceans relatively rapidly.

If all of the estimated recoverable reserves of coal, oil, and natural gas were burnt, 16 trillion tons of carbon dioxide would be produced. If all of that remained in the atmosphere, and assuming that we have a 4°F rise per doubling of CO_2 content, a 25°F rise in the average global temperature would result! But we have seen that in fact only about 40 per cent of the CO_2 is likely to stay in the atmosphere, and therefore, if all of those fuel reserves were combusted we would expect a 10°F rise in temperature. This would be an enormous rise in the average temperature of the earth's surface.

This number is probably not very realistic; I don't think anyone expects that all the recoverable reserves will be utilized. But if we look at the rate at which use of carbon fuels is increasing, and try to estimate realistically about where it will peak out as various other kinds of energy take over, we can arrive at an estimate of total carbon fuel use by the year 2050. The conclusion based on various expert projections for use of fossil fuels is that by 2050 we will have consumed about 80 per cent of all of the estimated recoverable oil reserves and just about all of the natural gas, and about 30 per cent of the estimated recoverable coal reserves. That much fuel consumption will result in a doubling of the CO_2 level. In other words, by 2050 there will be just about a doubling of the carbon dioxide content of the atmosphere, which will result in a 4°F rise in temperature, if these estimates are accurate.

The next question we must ask is: What does a 4°F rise in average global temperature mean? To get some feeling for this question we must look at the data from paleoclimatological studies involving the evidence of past climates. On the basis of various physical data, it has been possible to estimate the temperatures which prevailed at various times. The so-called *climatic optimun*, which occurred somewhere between 4000 B.C. and 2000 B.C., is a particularly interesting period, during which the climate was much warmer. It has been estimated that Arctic temperatures were as much as 4°F warmer than at present. And it is also believed by many experts that there was no permanent Arctic ice cap—that the Arctic ice was completely melted except for short periods during the winter. In agreement with this, theoretical studies with respect to the Arctic indicate that only a small change in temperature is required to completely melt the Arctic ice.

Since Arctic ice is floating, melting of the north polar ice cap would not result in a substantial change in the water level of the oceans. It would, however, be likely to have very profound effects on the distribution of ocean currents, which in turn could result in very different kinds of weather over much of the land mass in the Northern Hemisphere. It is just this land mass which has until now been the major source of food production for man. The melting of the north polar ice could therefore present a dangerous prospect, even though we don't know exactly what the outcome might be. There have been some calculations and estimates on the part of climatologists about this. For example, one expert contends that such an occurrence will result in a very arid climate through much of the temperate zone.

Climatologists agree that a 4°F rise in average global temperature would result in a very substantial melting of glaciers and the Greenland icecap and of the Antarctic icecap. To what extent melting would occur, and at what rate, is, however, not at all clear. If all the ice were to melt, the average ocean levels on earth would rise somewhere between 200 and 400 feet. Clearly, melting of all of this ice would be disastrous for many millions of people who live in heavily populated areas on the coasts. Even a ten or 15 foot rise in sea level would be disastrous.

We don't know enough about the factors which control global climate to know whether climatic changes of our own making might not trigger other, more substantial, climatic change. For example, melting of glaciers would reduce the amount of snow cover on the surface of the earth, averaged over the entire year. This would decrease the earth's albedo, the fraction of solar radiation reflected back into space. Ice and snow reflect a very large fraction of radiation back into space. Open water, soil, and rocks do not. But if a larger fraction of the sun's radiation were retained on earth, the effect would be an even larger degree of warming. As another example, warming the oceans would result in loss of carbon dioxide from them, since carbon dioxide is less soluble in warm than in cool water. ·This is not as large an effect as one might imagine. The estimates are that a 2°F rise in ocean temperature would result in about a 6 per cent increase of atmospheric carbon dioxide. Warming of the oceans therefore has the effect of amplifying slightly the effect of the added carbon dioxide.

It is clear from all this that man's additions of carbon dioxide to the atmosphere have the potential for creating a massive disaster, and it certainly is a problem that requires continued attention on the part of researchers. It is not at all obvious that we have an adequate model for carbon dioxide distribution and temperature in the ocean-atmosphere system. There is a need for more complex models, for which larger computers are required. But the data obtained from calculations so far seem to be reliable in the sense that they are not critically dependent on slight changes made in the model.

Because plants convert carbon dioxide to plant tissue in a process that begins with photosynthesis an increase in atmospheric CO_2 would undoubtedly result in increased plant growth. It is occasionally suggested that this might be a means by which excess CO_2 could be removed from the atmosphere, but a substantial fraction of CO_2 could not be taken from the atmosphere by this means. Plants eventually die, and in their decomposition CO_2 is returned to the atmosphere. Since the biomass contains a relatively small proportion of CO_2 in the first place, it seems clear that it could not store more than a fraction of the excess CO_2 being added to the environment.

PARTICLES IN THE ATMOSPHERE

Particulate matter may have the effect of increasing the earth's albedo. By particulate matter I mean particles of very small size which remain suspended in the atmosphere as an aerosol for a long time. That, in general, means particles on the order of 1 micron in diameter or smaller. The smoke that comes out of the local power plant stack consists of some particles which are that small, but it is made up mostly of the big, chunky black kind that soon come down on the surrounding neighborhood. These larger particles are not very important in terms of global climate, although they can be influential in determining a climate of public opinion. As a result of man's activities there has been a steady increase in the density of particles of the very small variety in the atmosphere. These particles have a number of possible effects. They can, for example, scatter incoming solar radiation back into space. This results in a cooling of the earth's climate, because that solar radiation doesn't contribute to the heat input. In one sense, then, particulate matter could cause a lowering of the earth's temperature.

The only data that really seem to bear on this area concern changes in the particle content of the atmosphere resulting from major volcanic eruption. When Krakatoa erupted in Java in 1888, there was an enormous input of volcanic ash into the stratosphere. The average particle size of those particles, as judged from light scattering studies done at that time, was on the order of one micron. The only solar observatory in operation in the world at that time was at Montpellier, in France. About six months after that explosion the dust finally arrived over France and caused a ten per cent decrease in the incoming solar radiation. The abnormally low levels were observed for about two years before the ash was effectively washed out of the atmosphere.

Particles can also produce other effects. For example, depending on the types of particles, they may be important in nucleating cloud formation. Stratospheric particles which nucleate clouds will produce cirrus type ice crystal clouds. Measurements indicate that high ice crystal clouds have a tendency to let solar radiation through—they have a low reflectivity toward solar radiation. They have a much higher reflectivity toward infrared radiation coming upward from earth. Furthermore, since they are in the stratosphere they are very cold clouds, and so are not very good black body radiators out into space. These clouds therefore tend to keep the earth's radiation in. They therefore may have the effect of warming the earth slightly, whereas lower-lying clouds may have the effect of cooling the earth's surface. All of this is to say that the effect of particulate matter is not clear. It is not at all certain whether their effect is to heat or to cool the earth.

One often reads the following argument in the papers, and in discussions of climatic trends: Since 1940 the earth has cooled off about 0.4°F while man has been pumping carbon dioxide into the atmosphere. The fact that the earth is cooling off shows that increasing particulate matter must be responsible, since carbon dioxide works in the opposite direction. But one can calculate how much carbon dioxide has been added to the atmosphere since 1935. If one applies the 40 per cent correction, and then takes Manabe and Wetherald's 4°F factor, one concludes that the amount of CO_2 added since 1935 should have warmed up the earth 0.2°F. This is obviously a small contribution. As to why the earth has cooled slightly, there are some very interesting recent data which bear on this. American and Danish scientists have taken a core of ice from the Greenland icecap. This mile-long core is layered on an annual basis, somewhat similarly to the rings of a tree. Measurements of the isotope ratio of ^{18}O to ^{16}O were made for various layers of the ice. This ratio is very sensitively dependent upon the temperature in the atmosphere at the instant the ice was deposited from the vapor. Although the isotope ratio doesn't give the temperature in degrees, it provides a *relative* measure of temperature change. This work shows the presence of more or less regular temperature variations, over a small range, extending back over the past 1000 years. The present cooling trend is a smooth part of this pattern of temperature variation. We do not understand what factors are responsible for the variations, but, whatever the causes, fluctuations of a few tenths of a degree Fahrenheit are quite normal. The carbon dioxide effect has not until now been very large; it hasn't been bigger than the natural fluctuations due to other influences. But in the next 80 years, man might add a 4°F perturbation; I suggest this will pretty much swamp the relatively minor effects which these measurements reflect.

ENERGY GENERATION

Finally, man can affect the average global temperature by generating heat at the surface of the earth. Although man is not yet competing with the sun on a global basis, he is capable of heating up the environment in local regions. For example, in the year 2000, in the region extending from Boston to Washington, D. C. on the eastern seaboard of the United States, the energy dissipation from man's activities in the wintertime will be about 50 per cent of the solar radiation at the ground level. It will be about 20 or 30 per cent of the solar radiation at ground level in the summertime. We can expect substantial changes in regional climate as a result of these high energy dissipation densities in the highly industrialized nations.

Extrapolating further into the future we can ask at what point man's energy producing activities begin to affect the global climate. Assuming—and this is a big assumption—that ways could be found to distribute energy dissipation uniformly over the planet's surface, the global rate of energy consumption could be about half of one per cent of the incoming solar energy input before material change in the average global temperature were noted. That one-half of one per cent would result in a 2°F rise in the average temperature on the surface of the earth. Even an increase of this magnitude might not be safe. It certainly represents the upper limit. To show what that number means, suppose there were a population on earth of eight billion people. Then the amount of energy just mentioned as the upper limit would allow a per capita energy consumption of about 70,000 watts.

The notion that there is no limit to the amount of energy that man can safely generate is absurd. The limits indicated could be exceeded only if the human race were to sacrifice much of the most habitable land mass. Today we are far from a per capita consumption of 70,000 watts. In the United States, the current per capita consumption, averaged over the entire population, is on the order of 12,000 to 14,000 watts. The world average per capita consumption is on the order of only 1500 watts. But energy use is doubling at a fairly rapid rate. In the United States the per capita energy consumption is doubling every 40 years, and for the world as a whole it doubles about every 25 years. In another couple of centuries, man could very well arrive at the ultimate limit in his capacity to generate energy.

SUGGESTED READING

Brown, T. L.: Energy and the Environment, Columbus, C. E. Merrill Publishing Co., 1971.

Man's Impact on the Global Environment, Cambridge, The MIT Press, 1970.

MOUSE OR MONSTER?

The Automobile as a Contribution to Pollution

Phillip S. Myers

Emissions from automobiles must be discussed in terms of pollution as an entity. Why have we suddenly become interested in pollution? How do we define pollution? At what rate is man putting pollutants in the atmosphere in comparison with the rate at which nature is doing so? What contribution is the automobile making towards polluting the atmosphere, and what has been done to reduce this contribution?

Pollution has become a problem simply because we are all polluters and each of us is polluting too much. Figure 1 shows a plot of the population of the earth as a function of time. Note that the population scale is not linear, but logarithmic—it rises in leaps of one-tenth, one, ten, etc. Note that despite the logarithmic scale, the slope of the curve is increasing. Those of you who are familiar with logarithmic scales know that an increase in slope on a logarithmic scale means that things are happening in a hurry! Clearly, the population of the earth is increasing dramatically.

With the dramatic increase in total population the per capita pollution is also increasing. Although there is no precise criterion of pollution, the best single index is per capita energy consumption. In generating energy we produce pollution. In utilizing energy to produce automobiles, refrigerators, and other consumer goods, we produce more pollution. Finally, we must get rid of the "remains" after we have made the product and it has served its purpose, and this produces additional pollution. Figure 2 is a plot of energy consumption per

53

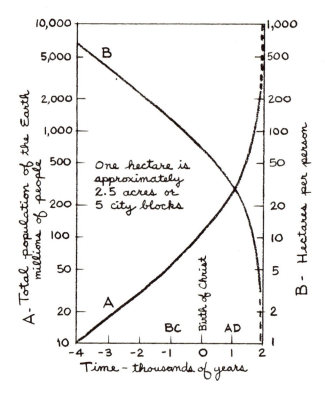

Figure 1: Population and area per person during the past six thousand years.

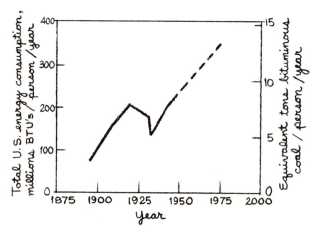

Figure 2: Energy use in The United States.

person, in the United States, for approximately the last 100 years. Per capita energy use has clearly been increasing steadily. Figure 3 shows

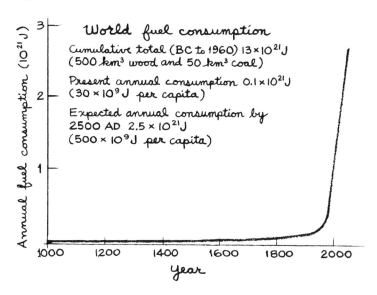

Figure 3: World-wide energy consumption.

the total world-wide energy consumption as a function of time. Again, the curve is going up very sharply.

What is a pollutant? How do we tell the good guys from the bad guys? With air pollution, we do this by determining if the effect of a suspected pollutant is detrimental to humans. Figure 4 lists several pollutants and the objectionable effect of each. The first pollutant listed is unburned gasoline (unburned hydrocarbon). This pollutant can have an objectionable odor, as for example one notices when driving along behind a diesel-powered truck or bus. There is, in addition, a potential for induced cancer, although this seems to be relatively small.

Unburned hydrocarbons also contribute to photochemical smog. We must make a distinction here between smog and photochemical smog; the latter requires four ingredients: sunlight, unburned hydrocarbon, oxygen, and oxides of nitrogen. This combination can produce

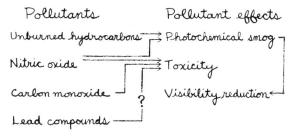

Figure: 4: Emissions and their effects from a spark-ignition gasoline engine.

the burning sensation in the eyes and the irritating sensation in the nose observed in photochemical smog areas such as Los Angeles. As the name implies, smog is a combination of smoke and fog. In general, the smoke in smog contains sulfur dioxide. Smog is really a combination of sulfur dioxide and fog, as distinguished from photochemical smog.

Oxides of nitrogen are another pollutant. As previously indicated, oxides of nitrogen are among the necessary ingredients for photochemical smog. Oxides of nitrogen are also toxic in their own right.

Carbon monoxide is another pollutant well known as a toxic agent.

Sulfur dioxide, produced mainly from burning of coal, is another toxic pollutant. A good bit of the sulfur dioxide put into the atmosphere combines with other materials and ends up as particulate matter. Particulates cause visibility reduction as well as lung damage.

Let us now look at the relative rates at which man and nature are pouring these pollutants into the atmosphere. Nature has always been pouring pollutants into the atmosphere. However, nature has also always been simultaneously destroying these pollutants. Thus the levels of pollutants in the atmosphere result from a balance between the rates at which they are added by one set of mechanisms and removed by another set. Man's activities affect this equilibrium, and we should therefore compare the rates of natural and man-made additions of pollutants. Figure 5 shows a typical mass rate balance. In the upper left

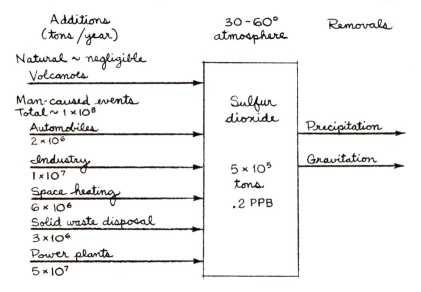

Figure 5: Mass rate balance for sulfur dioxide.

we see the rate at which nature has been adding material via natural events. Note that the rate is in tons per year. The center of the graph shows the amount in tons estimated to be in the atmosphere and the middle right shows the amount that man is putting in.

For particulate matter, about 10^8 tons per year are added via natural events (Figure 6). Man is putting particulates into the atmosphere at about the same rate -10^8 tons per year. I estimate that there

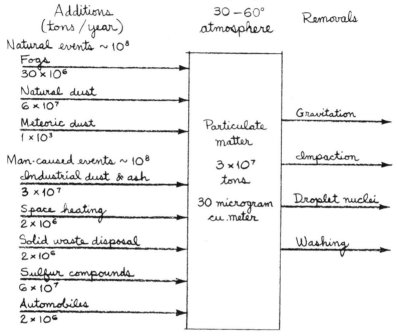

Figure 6: Mass rate balance for particulate matter.

are about three times 10^7 (about one-third as much) in the atmosphere. As shown on the right side of the figure, particulate matter is removed from the atmospheric environment mainly by settling out and by forming droplet nuclei in rain.

Natural events produce a total quantity of about 0.2 x 10^8 tons of carbon monoxide annually, while man-caused events result in about 2 x 10^8 tons, or about ten times as much. However, estimates of the amount of naturally occurring CO in the atmosphere are undergoing revision at present. It appears that the natural production of CO is really much higher than previously thought. Figure 7 lists some of the effects of carbon monoxide, which is, of course, a toxic substance, while Table I shows some of the concentrations of carbon monoxide to which we are exposed. The oxygen-carrying function of blood depends on the affinity of hemoglobin for oxygen. However, hemoglobin has a greater

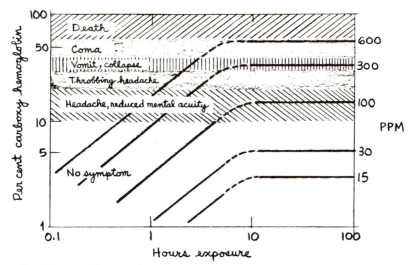

Figure 7: Toxic effects of carbon monoxide.

affinity for carbon monoxide than oxygen. Figure 7 displays a plot of time versus per cent carboxyhemoglobin. The left scale shows the percentage of hemoglobin occupied by carbon monoxide rather than by oxygen. You can see, for example, that if a person were exposed to an atmosphere containing 100 parts CO per million, after a period of 8 to

TABLE 1
Measured CO Concentrations

Urban Areas

> 38 ppm - 1 hour
>
> 27 ppm - 8 hours
>
> 17 ppm - 24 hours

Moving Vehicles

> Peak: 75 ppm - 5 min.
>
> Median: 60 ppm

Cigarette Smoke

> 42,000

10 hours a little better than 10 per cent of the hemoglobin in his blood would be occupied by carbon monoxide, (10% carboxyhemoglobin) rather than by oxygen.

The region of the graph of particular interest is the area of 15–30 ppm. There is controversial evidence for a detectable effect at this low concentration. For example, there is some indication that a person exposed to atmospheres having 15–30 ppm of CO cannot add a list of figures quite as rapidly or accurately as he can at lower concentrations of CO. It is noteworthy that moderate to heavy smokers carry about five per cent carboxyhemoglobin in their blood in the latter part of the day.

Table I shows some of the concentrations of CO that one is normally exposed to. In urban areas exposures may run on order of 40 ppm for the duration of an hour, and to considerably higher concentrations for shorter periods. A recent study in Madison, Wisconsin, for example, has shown momentary concentrations as high as 150 ppm. Over an eight-hour period, however, the concentration averages only 27 ppm. For a 24 hour period the average is 17 ppm. The driver of a moving vehicle in traffic may be exposed to 60–75 ppm. The concentration of CO in cigarette smoke, on the other hand, is on the order of 42,000 ppm! How excited should we get about carbon monoxide from cars if people voluntarily expose themselves to these extraordinarily high concentrations?

In the case of the oxides of nitrogen, natural events put in about 2×10^8 tons per year; man-caused events add about 5×10^7 or about one-quarter as much (Figure 8). However, these data are on a global basis. Figure 9 shows some data on a local basis. Note that in Los Angeles natural processes are putting in around 10,000 tons per year whereas man-caused events are putting in around 350,000 tons per year, about 35 times as much. It's no wonder that Los Angeles has a problem with oxides of nitrogen.

Nature adds very little sulfur dioxide to the atmosphere. Most of what is put into the atmosphere comes from man, primarily as a result of burning coal with sulfur in it. There is some sulfur in fuel oil and gasoline but most of that is taken out during the refining process.

One of the other pollutants that has been in the headlines recently is lead. You will remember that lead is put in gasoline in order to improve its combustion characteristics. Combustion in a car engine is very rapid, but not quite rapid enough to be called an explosion. The combustion flame starts at the spark plug. The flame front progresses across the combustion chamber in a fast but orderly way. However, the gasoline-air mixture is quite reactive chemically. In addition, the last part of the mixture to burn is compressed first by the piston and later

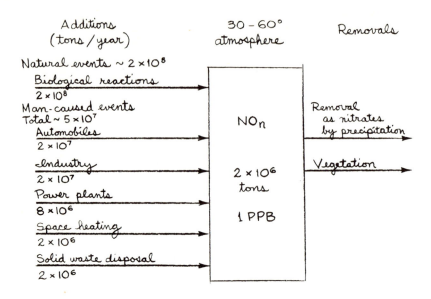

Figure 8: Mass rate balance for oxides of nitrogen.

by the early combustion. Eventually the highly reactive air-fuel mixture reaches a point at which it truly does explode, producing "ping" or "knock".

Experimentally it has been found that if we put some lead in the gasoline the unburned air-fuel mixture will burn more slowly and more regularly. Unfortunately we don't know exactly the mechanism by which lead operates in this process.

Although we still fundamentally don't know the details of what goes on during combustion we do know that if we add lead it reduces knock in an engine and we can use fuel more efficiently—get more miles per gallon. Of course we also know that at the same time there is a possibility of lead adversely affecting people, since lead is a poison. Figure 10 shows a mass balance for the lead that is put in an automobile gas tank. Roughly 40 per cent goes out the exhaust pipe in

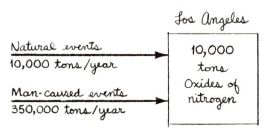

Figure 9: Local mass rule balance for oxides of nitrogen in the Los Angeles basin.

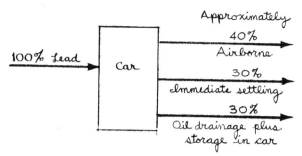

Figure 10: Distribution of lead emissions.

particles so small that they remain airborne. Another 30 per cent comes out in the form of considerably larger particles and settles down as dust on the street or in the close vicinity of the street or highway. The remaining 30 per cent either remains in the combustion chamber or exhaust system of the car or goes into the lubricating system and is drained out with the oil.

Figure 11 shows a mass rate balance for lead for us as individuals. We take in lead via the air that we breathe, and, secondly, via the digestive tract—from food and water. The amount of lead we ingest via food and water is some twenty or thirty times that brought in via the air. This isn't quite the entire story, because more of the lead that enters the respiratory system is absorbed than that which comes in via the digestive tract. Since the amount of lead that we take in via food and water seems to be the controlling factor in determining lead

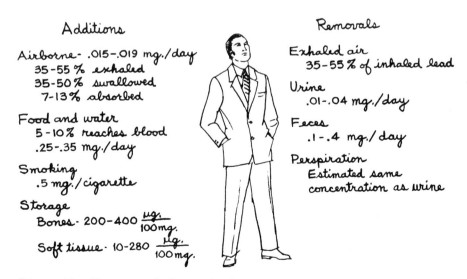

Figure 11: Mass rate balance for human exchange of lead.

levels in the body, I have come to the conclusion that we need not take lead out of gasoline because of possible damage to us as individuals. I will point out later on, however, that we may wish to take it out because it does affect exhaust control systems which might be used on an automobile.

The final mass rate balance is for unburned hydrocarbons—unburned gasolines. Again, not very good data are available. The data in Figure 12 are very rough estimates. Most of the unburned hydrocarbons produced in nature are in the form of natural gas. There is much more "swamp gas" or methane than most people realize. Also, the smell of the pine forest most of us like so well is really the smell of hydrocarbons.

What is the contribution of the automobile to our pollution problem? Man is beginning to dump materials into the atmosphere at a rate that is significant with respect to the rate which nature adds those same pollutants. Clearly the automobile is a contributor, especially on a mass basis. There is some question, however, whether we should simply weigh pollution contributions or whether we should not also consider toxicity. I will show you data from both standpoints.

Figure 13 shows the contribution of the automobile on a mass basis in millions of tons per year. Comparing the bar graph for the transportation industry and that for all other industry grouped together, we can see that the contribution of the automobile is about equal to

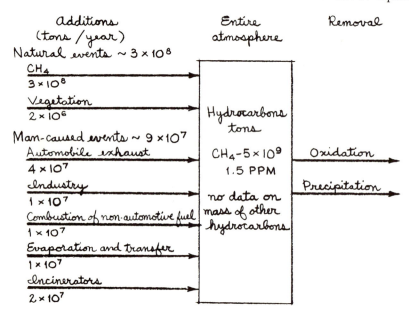

Figure 12: Mass rate balance for hydrocarbons.

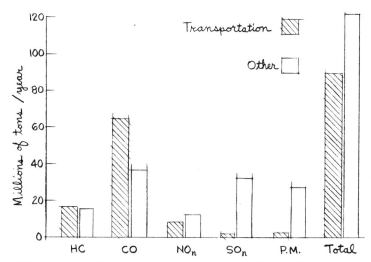

Figure 13: Automobile emissions by weight (H. E. W. data for 1968).

that of all other industry. The automobile puts out roughly 50 per cent more carbon monoxide and about the same amount of oxides of nitrogen as does all other industry. It puts out very little sulfur dioxide and very little particulate matter in comparison with other industries. The last two bars on the right hand side show the total; the automobile, on a mass basis, emits about 40 per cent of the total pollution in the atmosphere.

I believe, however, that it is wrong to equate a pound of sugar and a pound of arsenic and that one should look at the problem on a combined mass and toxicity basis. There can be arguments, of course, as to how the correction for toxicity is to be made.

Figure 14 shows the bars of Figure 13, weighted according to the air quality standards set up by the State of California. The logic is that the lower the permissible standard, the more toxic the material must be. On a toxicity basis the hydrocarbons do not contribute much, carbon monoxide is fairly negligible, oxides of nitrogen are not very important, whereas sulfur dioxide and particulate matter are quite important. On a combined mass-toxicity basis the automobile contribution is on the order of 12 to 15 per cent. This, in my opinion, represents a more realistic assessment of the automobile's contribution to pollution. In any event the automobile is a significant polluter and we should be doing what we can to reduce its contribution.

Figure 15 shows various sources of emission from a car and their relative magnitudes. You will note that some of the gasoline vaporizing from the tank escapes to the atmosphere. This contributes roughly 10 per cent of the total emissions. The same thing happens with the

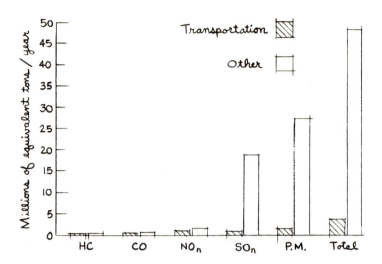

Figure 14: *United States air pollution displayed on a relative-effect basis. Pollutant weights are adjusted to the same effect level as that of particulate matter.*

Automotive sources of air pollution

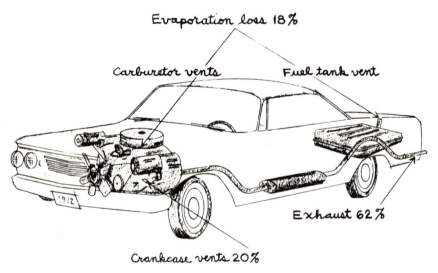

Figure 15: *Automotive sources of air pollution.*

carburetor, particularly when the car is stopped on a warm day with the engine hot. Gasoline is vaporized from the carburetor, contributing roughly 10 per cent of the emissions from the car. Some of the gases in the combustion chamber leak by the piston, and come out the crankcase vent contributing about 20 per cent to the emissions. Exhaust gases make up the remaining 60 per cent of the car's total contribution to pollution.

Beginning in 1964, all cars manufactured in the United States had to have a device to control crankcase pollution. This device (Figure 16) takes clean filtered air in through the air cleaner, leads it down into

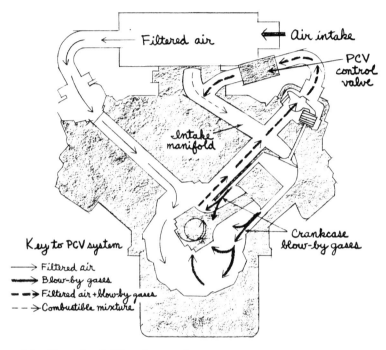

Figure 16: How the PCV valve works.

the crankcase and back up thru the positive crankcase ventilation (PCV) valve. The outlet from the PCV control valve goes to the inlet manifold; thus crankcase emissions are burnt in the combustion chamber. If this system is properly maintained it essentially eliminates crankcase emissions. The PCV valve, however, has a difficult life, since it has a rather messy mixture flowing over it. If you are a good ecologist, you will clean or replace your PCV valve every six months or so in order not to pollute the atmosphere. It is also good economics to clean or replace the PCV valve, because the gases are quite corrosive. If the PCV valve gets clogged up the gases are not taken out of the crankcase as intended, and the life of the engine is shortened.

In 1970 for cars manufactured for use in California, and in 1971 on a nation-wide basis, controls were put on fuel evaporation. Figure 17 shows how these controls operate. Fuel vapors escaping from the tank

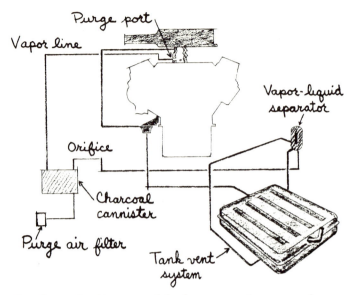

Figure 17: A schematic diagram of fuel evaporation controls.

or from the carburetor are led to a charcoal cannister. Charcoal has the ability to adsorb hydrocarbon vapors. When the car is not operating and if fuel is vaporizing, these vapors are absorbed by the charcoal. When the car is started air is automatically drawn over the charcoal. The adsorbed fuel vapors are drawn off by this air and taken into the engine where they are burned. It appears that about 90 per cent of the fuel that is vaporized is controlled in this way.

This leaves the exhaust gases as the remaining source of pollutants. In the cylinder (Figure 18) a spark starts a flame burning across the combustion chamber. When the flame gets quite close to the cylinder wall the relatively cold cylinder wall "quenches" the flame so it doesn't burn quite all the way to the wall. There is, therefore, a thin quench layer of a few thousandths of an inch of unburned fuel and air next to the cylinder wall. When the piston comes up and pushes out the exhaust gases, it scrapes off the quench layer and pushes it out the exhaust along with the other gases. Because the other gases are hot, about two-thirds of the relatively cool air-fuel mixture is burnt in the exhaust. The other one-third comes out in a relatively unburned state.

The two other major pollutants formed in the combustion chamber are carbon monoxide and oxides of nitrogen. These seem to be formed in the center of the cylinder, in what is called the bulk gas.

Carbon monoxide formation is primarily a result of oxygen deficiency. A plot of carbon monoxide content as a function of air/fuel ratio produces a very nice correlation, as shown in Figure 19. The

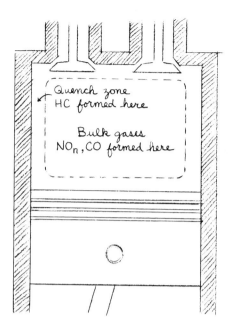

Figure 18: Locales of emission formation in the cylinder of a gasoline engine.

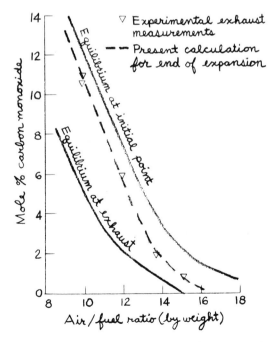

Figure 19: Carbon monoxide formation as a function of air-fuel ratio.

chemically correct mixture is around 15½ pounds of air per pound of fuel. On the fuel-rich side (oxygen deficiency), there is considerable carbon monoxide production, but when on the lean side (oxygen surplus) there is very little carbon monoxide. Notice that the experimental values are between what you would anticipate if you looked at equilibrium at the highest temperature in the cylinder and if you looked at equilibrium at the lowest temperature in the cylinder. Thus the actual value is determined partially by chemical kinetics.

Oxides of nitrogen, the second pollutant of combustion, are not thermodynamically stable at room temperature, but they are stable at the high temperatures which prevail when they are formed. Chemical kinetics are definitely dominant in determining the actual concentration of oxides of nitrogen. It takes time to form the oxides of nitrogen after the flame has passed through the mixture. Also, once the oxides are formed, it takes time to destroy them. In general, however, when the peak temperature increases the concentration of oxides of nitrogen increases considerably.

Figure 20 illustrates the details of what happens. The plot of temperature versus time is characteristic of the temperature history in the cylinder of an engine. Let us next look at what happens to the oxides of nitrogen. If chemical equilibrium were established at all times production of oxides of nitrogen would have gone up quite rapidly as the temperature increased. However, because the chemical reactions lag behind the temperature rise, the actual formation of the oxides lags behind, and by the time it begins to catch up, the temperature has begun to drop. As the temperature drops further, the rates of destruction are slowed down so the oxides of nitrogen remain at a relatively high

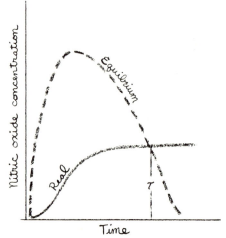

Figure 20: Nitrogen oxide formation.

value. The net result is that chemical kinetics determines almost exclusively the amount of nitrogen oxides formed in the exhaust. Again,
from a practical standpoint, almost anything we do to increase the peak
temperature tends to increase the concentrations of nitrogen oxides.

Recall that there is a chemically correct air-fuel mixture, which
corresponds to the mark S on the plot of pollutants versus air/fuel
ratio by (Figure 21). Running on the rich side (excess fuel) produces
high concentrations of carbon monoxide and hydrocarbons. Running on
the lean side (deficiency of fuel) decreases the hydrocarbon and carbon
monoxide levels, but increases the amount of oxides of nitrogen. Thus
the automobile engineer, to a certain extent, is in a dilemma. Is he
going to set the carburetor to run rich and pollute with carbon monoxide
and hydrocarbons, or is he going to set it lean and pollute with oxides
of nitrogen?

On the other hand, another aspect of the question must be considered, driveability. Suppose you were to take a car to a level road
with no wind. Suppose we had some way of varying the air/fuel ratio
as you drive down the road holding your foot steady on the accelerator
pedal. If we started with the chemically correct mixture and went toward the rich side, we could go quite far before anything would happen.
Eventually, though, the car would begin to speed up and slow down—to
surge. We do not completely understand exactly why this happens. It
is combination of combustion and the operation of the carburetor and
intake manifold; nevertheless, it happens. If we go toward the lean
side we do not get very far beyond the chemically correct ratio until a

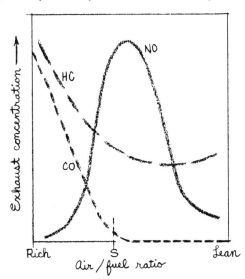

Figure 21: The effect of the air/fuel ratio on emissions.

similar effect occurs. Consequently manufactures have tended to set
the carburetors on the rich side in order to provide good driveability.
In recent years, however, because of the emphasis on pollutants, the
carburetor settings have been moving more towards the lean side. The
hydrocarbon and carbon monoxide emissions have thus gone down but
the oxides of nitrogen have, if anything, tended to increase.

I have already indicated that two-thirds of the hydrocarbons exhausted from the cylinder are burned in the exhaust system. Fundamentally, this is the method that has been used to control hydrocarbons
and carbon monoxide so far. A number of things have been done to
improve combustion in the exhaust system. First, a higher-temperature
thermostat causes the engine to operate at a higher temperature. Retarding the timing of the spark has been found to make the exhaust-gas
temperature higher. These changes have helped in decreasing hydrocarbon and carbon monoxide emission. In general, however, such
expedients have decreased fuel economy on the order of 10 or 15 per
cent. We get fewer miles per gallon and are thus using up more of a
relatively scarce resource.

Of course we can go even further in terms of destroying the hydrocarbon and carbon monoxide in the exhaust. It would help to better
insulate the exhaust system, producing what is called a thermal reactor. But how do you produce at reasonable costs an exhaust system
that will survive at temperatures on the order of 1800°F? What happens
to the temperature of the thermal reactor when a spark plug misfires and
the resulting unburned fuel is consumed in the reactor?

An alternative approach, that will quite probably be used, is to put
a catalytic muffler in the exhaust system. A catalyst serves the same
purpose as a shotgun at a wedding: it doesn't take part in the process
but it speeds things up. In a catalytic muffler the temperature required
for complete oxidation of hydrocarbon and carbon is lowered. Most of
the really good oxidation catalysts used at present are noble metals,
platinum for example, and are expensive and scarce. Although some
of the cheaper metals now appear to have promise, they have not yet
been introduced. In addition, the catalyst has a pretty rough life; it is
repeatedly heated and cooled in addition to being shaken by car motion.
After a time the catalyst may come out the tail pipe as particulate
matter. There is also the problem of the time needed for the catalyst
to warm up. In the test cycle used for testing emissions, the car is
started up cold. It takes a little time for the catalyst to warm up and
act. Thus, if the engine and catalyst warm up slowly all the hydrocarbons permitted by test regulations may have been put out before the
catalyst is warm and active. It is clear that there are real difficulties
in meeting the 1975 exhaust emission standards.

Because lead tends to poison the catalysts which presently seem most promising there is a fundamental need for taking lead out of gasoline if we are to use catalytic mufflers. Other trace ingredients which may poison catalysts may also need to be removed for (or not added to) gasoline.

It is interesting to look at what we have accomplished and what it has cost, how much farther we might go, and how much that might cost. The graph is Figure 22 shows hydrocarbon emission in grams per mile *versus* relative power plant cost. I have set the cost of an uncontrolled engine as one unit. Automobile pollutants are expressed today in terms of grams per mile. Imagine that a bag is tied to the tailpipe of your car that would let everything through but the hydrocarbons. The bag would catch the hydrocarbons coming out the exhaust during a one-mile drive, involving acceleration, deceleration, etc. The weight of the material in the bag would be the grams of hydrocarbons per mile. In 1960, before we started using emission controls, a car put out on the order of 19 grams per mile. By definition this design of engine has one unit of cost. In 1964 crankcase controls were applied. This brought hydrocarbons down to something like 15 grams per mile at a few per cent increase in the cost of the engine. In 1968 exhaust controls were added to crankcase controls. The combination reduced hydrocarbon emissions to between 7 and 8 grams per mile at about a 10 per cent increase in engine cost. In 1971 fuel evaporative controls were added and emissions came down to 2.2 grams per mile, with a total cost increase of something like 15 per cent. The 1975 standards may be something like a quarter of a gram per mile on this scale (the actual number

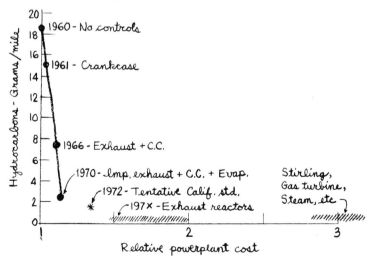

Figure 22: The economics of hydrocarbon reduction.

is higher but on a different scale). This is a very, very low standard and represents a tremendous reduction. These low requirements will probably be met by either the thermal reactor or the catalytic muffler. The best estimates are that this will cause the cost of the engine to increase to 150 to 200 per cent of the cost of the 1960 engine.

On the far right hand side of Figure 22 are shown steam engines, gas turbines, and Stirling engines—other types of power plants. It is true that these competitive power plants can achieve low hydrocarbon emissions. However, the best estimate is that they will cost between two and three times as much as the uncontrolled engine, which explains the general lack of enthusiasm for these alternative power sources.

A plot for carbon monoxide similar to that in Figure 22 would show that we have reduced carbon monoxide by about 60 per cent. However, we have increased rather than decreased the oxides of nitrogen except for the last two or three years. Retarding the spark a bit has lowered the gas temperature and thus the oxides of nitrogen. However, this means lower gas mileage.

To meet the 1975 standards, I'm reasonably sure that it will be necessary to bring some of the exhaust gases into the carburetor along with the air, because this will serve as an inert diluent to hold down the peak gas temperature, and in turn to hold down the oxides of nitrogen. This, however, will also decrease the power output of the engine.

What is the effect of all of these controls on the quality of the atmosphere? Figure 23 shows a plot of the mass of material put into the atmosphere by the automobile in tons per year as a function of time. The amount of material has been going up consistently. This simply reflects the fact that there are more automobiles each year and that each automobile is being driven slightly more. The dotted line is an

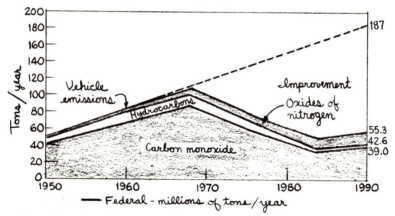

Figure 23: Actual and projected improvements in automotive emissions in the United States.

extrapolation of what would have happened if no controls had been present. The amounts that have actually been placed into the atmosphere are shown in the lower curve. You can see a slight change in curvature beginning in 1961 and a sharper change beginning in 1968 when exhaust controls began. These controls, however, apply only to new cars; old cars are still being used. Thus the amount of pollutant actually going into the atmosphere represents the combined effect of the new and the old cars. Because old cars are being junked the curve decreases until sometime around 1980. At that time, unless something else is done, the curve will start back up again.

These considerations indicate that our society has real problems in setting technological standards. How do we balance the many conflicting parameters that should be considered in a policy-making decision? It is, I think, one of the facts of life that one receives an ever smaller return for increased technological investment. As an example, it didn't cost very much to decrease hydrocarbons by 50 per cent, but a second reduction of 50 per cent will cost much more than the first. The second consideration is human misery and death. Clearly if we keep on polluting the air we are going to have many more serious air pollution incidents and an increased mortality rate among people in marginal health. The relationship between air quality and human misery must be part of our considerations. We must combine all these factors to determine an optimal cost-benefit relationship which embraces not only technological considerations but basic human values as well.

SUGGESTED READING

Myers, P. S., Automobile Emissions — A Study in Environmental Benefits Versus Technological Costs, Soc. of Automotive Engineers Transactions, S. A. E. Paper 700182, 1970.

Myers, P. S., Uyehara, O. A., and Newhall, H. K., The ABC's of Engine Exhaust Emissions, Soc. of Automotive Engineers Transactions, S. A. E. Paper 710481, 1971.

TO WEED OR NOT TO WEED

Herbicides

Julius E. Johnson

Crop yields and the general productivity of agriculture over the centuries remained constant until quite recently. In Great Britain, historical records dating from the twelfth century indicate yields of about 500 pounds of wheat per acre in the year 1100. By the year 1900, yields were in the range of 1500 pounds per acre; by 1930, 2000 pounds; and by 1960, 4000 pounds. The increase in yield between 1930 and 1960 is typical of other improvements in agriculture. Since 1870, United States yields of wheat, oats, barley, corn, and cotton have improved substantially, as shown in Table 1. Champaign-Urbana is in the center of one of the best crop yielding areas, where it is not uncommon to attain yields of 150 to 200 bushels of corn per acre.

TABLE 1
**Approximate Yield Per Acre of Some
Major Crops in the U.S. 1870 - 1969**

CROP	MEASURE	1870	1940	1969
CORN	Bushels	29	28	84
WHEAT	Bushels	12	15	33
OATS	Bushels	26	35	53
BARLEY	Bushels	22	23	44
COTTON	Pounds	208	252	436

Expressed another way, about 328 million fewer acres are needed today to produce the same total yield that was produced in 1940.

The United States now produces over one-half the world production of corn and two-thirds of the soybeans. These are our most important export crops today and their acceptance in the world market is increasing. We provide better than 90 per cent of the soybeans exported in the world market; and, of course, different types of soybean meal are an inexpensive source of protein and are used extensively in poultry and swine feeds. Much of this increased productivity is the result of improved agricultural technology.

FARM LABOR REQUIREMENT

Another important change resulting from the improved application of agricultural technology can be seen in the size of the farm labor force. Today 5 per cent of our population works on farms. In 1959, it was 10 per cent; in 1945, 25 per cent. This liberation of labor from the farm to industry has created not only great industrial development but also complex social problems. However, it is typical of a nation advancing in economic stature. Between 1945 and 1964 the fraction of the U. S. population on the land was 7 per cent; in Canada the figure was 11 per cent; in the Soviet Union, 39 per cent; in Mexico, 54 per cent; in India, 73 per cent; and in Thailand, 82 per cent. A large fraction of the population of the underdeveloped countries is occupied in the lower end of modern man's hierarchy of values. In the process of surviving, much time is spent in the planting, weeding, and harvesting of crops. And of all these chores, the weeding of crops usually consumes the most time and energy.

Why weed crops? The simple answer is that weeds are competitors. They compete for light. They compete for moisture. They compete for nutrients in the soil. They compete for space. Experiments to demonstrate competition between crops and weeds have been conducted by many investigators. One example focuses attention on the importance of competition for plant nutrients. In an unweeded field, the crop plants and the weeds from a given area were harvested and analyzed for total nutrient uptake from the soil. The weeds contained 1.6 times as much phosphorous, 2.5 times as much potassium, 7.6 times as much calcium, 3.3 times as much magnesium, and twice as much nitrogen as the crop forced to compete in the same plot of ground.

In underdeveloped countries, where the nutrient level of the land is often quite low, competition from weeds is a factor seriously limiting economic wellbeing. Disproportionate percentages of the people must spend inordinate amounts of time laboriously removing weeds from their crops in order to obtain any useful yields.

THE WEED PROBLEM

Now, let us turn our attention to the situation in the United States. Since Illinois is in the heart of the most productive cropping area for corn and soybeans, I will concentrate on weed control in these crops, but will also touch on another very different use of herbicides involving several leading compounds such as 2,4-D and 2,4,5-T. The latter has been a subject of controversy lately and I want to apprise you of certain points in that regard.

Weeds decrease yield. They steal from the farmer's time. They reduce land values. They increase costs of harvesting. Harvested crops infested with noxious weed seeds bring lower prices. Weeds limit the choice of crops that can be grown productively on many soils. If mechanical cultivation procedures are used to suppress weeds in the growing crop, the resultant root-pruning of crop plants often damages the crops. With drilled crops, such as small grains, tillage usually is not possible after crop emergence. Where rainfall and soil moisture are naturally limiting and weeds are rampant, there is practically no way to produce crops successfully. These are just some of the reasons that herbicides are needed.

There are some less obvious reasons. Good water management in irrigated areas is closely associated with weed control since water consumption by weeds can be very costly. Insects and plant diseases are harbored in weedy areas. For example, the wild carrot is a haven for the carrot weevil. Aphids live on mustard plants and spread to cabbage or cauliflower. Curly top, a virus disease problem in beets, is carried by an insect vector which lives on the weed Russian thistle. Over-wintering insects are protected from winter cold in weedy areas, which allows more of them to survive for the next season of crop depredation. Weeds can affect the quality of agricultural products. The disagreeable flavor of wild onion or wild garlic in milk usually occurs in spring or early summer when cows are turned out to pasture and vary their diet with onion or garlic, which are weed pests in the pastures. A sizeable fraction of our population suffers from allergies—a common allergy being sensitivity to ragweed. Poison ivy in recreational areas causes much discomfort and even serious illness to thousands of people each year.

How does the farmer look at weeds? The 1970 National Survey of Weed Losses in Soybeans reports that a median infestation may result in a loss of $8 to $22 per acre. If the infestation by weeds is heavy and uncontrolled, the loss may be $18 to $35 per acre. A so-called "disaster infestation" can cut the yield 35 to 100 per cent, and cause a dollar loss of $35 to $100 or more per acre, depending on the crop.

BIOLOGICAL CONTROL

The question of the efficacy of biological control often comes up in relation to the control of pests. Effective biological control of weeds has been limited to a few cases. To apply this method successfully, it is necessary to understand and adapt production practices to the insect life cycles. Once the food supply for the insect (the weed being controlled) has been reduced or eliminated by the insect, the insect population is in turn drastically reduced or eliminated. Hence complete or even adequate control of a troublesome weed pest is rarely possible, even though there are a few examples of successful biological control.

The prickly-pear cactus in Australia became a serious economic rangeland problem. Biologists discovered a moth in Argentina which attacks cactus, and this exogenous species was imported to Australia. The net result was virtual elimination of the prickly-pear cactus problem, with resulting starvation and die-off of the moth and a consequent, though moderate, repopulation by the prickly-pear. Then the population of the moth increased, followed by a die-off of the prickly-pear. This cycle was repeated until, finally, there was a stabilization of prickly-pear infestation at a level which was more tolerable than the original one.

In Hawaii, the thorny shrub lantana was controlled rather successfully by the introduction of a parasitic moth. In the western United States, St. Johnswort was in part controlled by the use of a leaf-eating beatle. Except for a few examples such as these, the success of biological control of weeds has been limited.

DEVELOPMENT OF CHEMICAL WEED CONTROL

A survey of Central Illinois farmers showed that weed problem as a whole is comprised of a series of problems with specific weeds. In both corn and soybeans, foxtails are considered the worst problem, and pigweed rates second. From first-hand observation of my brother-in-law's farm near Bement, I would concur that giant foxtail is a major problem. If this one particular weed is not controlled, he can suffer ruinous losses.

The history of weed control by chemical herbicides is mostly recent. H. L. Bolley, an agronomist in North Dakota, was interested in various inorganic salts for selective control of weeds in wheat. In 1908, he experimented with copper salts, sodium chloride, and chlorates. These salts were not very useful for selective weed control. Chlorates gained acceptance for overall vegetation control on railroad and industrial sites but were later supplanted by more effective herbicides. In 1941, R. Pokorny first synthesized 2,4-dichlorophenoxyacetic acid (2,4-D). It was tested for fungicidal and insecticidal properties and found to be inactive. Very interestingly, in those first laboratory observations, the formative effects of 2,4-D were not observed. One year later, A. E. Hitchcock and P. W. Zimmerman, studying various plant growth "hormones" discovered the plant growth effects of 2,4-D. In 1943, P. C. Marth and J. W. Mitchell, of the U. S. Department of Agriculture, selectively controlled dandelions in turf. C. L. Hammer and H. B. Tukey at Geneva, New York, first demonstrated the use of 2,4-D as a selective herbicide in crops. The preemergence herbicide concept was first developed by W. G. Templeman in 1945. These were the beginnings of very intensive research, in this country and abroad, into the chemical control of weeds.

The use of herbicides has grown rapidly in the United States. In 1966, 117 million acres were treated, increasing to about 154 million in 1970 when approximately 510 million dollars were spent for this type of weed control.

HERBICIDE TERMINOLOGY

Each herbicide has its specific mode of action. Furthermore, the time of the specific action must be matched with the growth cycle of various crop plants and weeds. Consider the situation of a weed seed in the soil. The seed germinates, the seedling emerges and grows, and the plant matures. The herbicide may be applied at various stages in this process of development. Herbicides that are active on the dormant seed are few. One of the most effective is a gas, methylbromide, which is toxic to weed seeds, provided the seeds are not too dry. Methylbromide is difficult to handle and is expensive to apply because the gas must be confined under a gas-proof cover. Its use is primarily on seed beds for starting high-value crops, such as ornamental plants or tobacco. After the cover is removed the gas dissipates and the treated soil can be planted with the desired seed or seedlings.

A *pre-emergence* herbicide, normally applied after planting a crop but before the crop seedlings emerge, is toxic to the newly germinating weed seeds, after the radicles have emerged. A *postemergence* herbicide is applied after weeds and crop emerge from the soil. Some herbicides are applied prior to planting and are mixed into the soil by tillage. This is called *preplant incorporation.*

I have used the terms selective and nonselective. For the control of dandelions in lawns 2,4-D is an example of a selective herbicide. A nonselective herbicide is used for general control of existing weedy vegetation. Railroad berms, parking lots, and fire control zones are areas where nonselective herbicides can be very useful. Chlorinated phenyl ureas represent one family of nonselective herbicides used for this purpose.

Contact herbicides are those which can be applied to burn the foliage. Petroleum oils and dinitrophenols are contact herbicides. Growth modifiers are another class of herbicides. These agents slow the growth of plants, without killing them, to reduce competition with the desired plant to a tolerable level.

Translocation, a term frequently used in connection with herbicides, means the movement of the herbicide—either from the roots, from the leaves, or from the bark or stem to other parts of a plant. A *systemic* herbicide is one which is translocated from one part of a plant to another part. Not all systemics translocate to the roots. Many systemic herbicides go up but not down. The term *soil sterilant* refers to a rather longlasting herbicide which provides weed control over an extended period of time.

Preplant, pre-emergence, and postemergence are terms related to time. Placement is also important. There is a *broadcast* treatment—overall treatment of a field or area. There is *band* treatment—application on a band, usually over the row in which crop seeds are planted. The remainder of the field, between the rows, is cultivated. Then there are *directed* and *spot* treatments. Directed sprays are used for weed control in row crops where over-the-top spraying is not adequately selective. Some of you are familiar with the use of drop nozzles to apply 2,4-D to the weeds in corn without getting the spray on the corn foliage. In Australia, eucalyptus is a common tree which overruns valuable rangeland. It can be controlled with spot treatment. For example, picloram, one of the newer herbicides, is very effective when applied in a basal application or as an injection. Directed spot treatment is used for the final control of patches of Canada thistle. Once the population of Canada thistle, or other perennial weed pest, has beed reduced by overall treatment or tillage, there often is no further need for overall broadcast spraying. The farmer can control the remaining plants economically by spot treating them.

HERBICIDE USE

A few statistics on the timing of herbicide use may be of interest. In one study, 19 per cent of corn farmers applied their herbicide ahead of planting, 29 per cent during planting, 28 per cent after planting, and 22 per cent before lay-by. If you have seen a corn planter rigged to plant corn, to place fertilizer and to apply herbicide all in one pass through the field, you have seen a technological break-through in application technique. There is an increasing trend toward herbicide application during planting to minimize the compaction of soil which results from each pass of heavy equipment through a field. 2,4-D is the herbicide most widely used after the corn emerges.

In the case of soybeans, growers have reported on use of herbicides as follows: 28 per cent preplant, 47 per cent during the planting operation, and 23 per cent after planting.

The question might be raised, "What does the farmer think about the value of herbicides?" Judging from what he observes in the field, and tempered by the profit motive, a cross-section of Illinois farmers concluded in 1970 that their weed control results in corn rated about 70 per cent good and 26 per cent fair. In the case of soybeans, they reported about 66 per cent good and about 28 per cent fair results (Table 2). Several factors are known to affect success with herbicides: dosage, soil type, timing, and weather (especially rainfall).

The cost to the farmer of different types of herbicides may be of interest. An inexpensive treatment is an overall application or a directed 2,4-D spray in corn, costing about 50 to 60 cents per acre for

TABLE 2
Average Effectiveness of Herbicide Treatment
Illinois 1970

	PER CENT [1]		
	POOR	FAIR	GOOD
CORN, Pre-emergence	4	26	70
CORN, Postemergence	4	27	69
SOYBEANS	6	28	66

[1]Data from questionnaires to 12,000 farmers. Thus, 66 to 70% of the farmers using herbicides reported good control, 26 to 28% fair control, and 4 to 6% poor control of weeds.

the herbicide. A more expensive treatment comprises a precombination of herbicides applied pre-emergence, costing in the neighborhood of 7 to 10 dollars per acre. The overall value received compared to the cost to the grower in today's farm economy is in the ratio of 4 to 1, four dollars of profit for each dollar expended for herbicide. In the case of fertilizers, a comparable ratio is about 2.5 to 1. These are national averages and will vary case by case and farm by farm. The most efficient growers achieve higher ratios because they pay attention to proper application of the best performance materials.

SOME HERBICIDES

There are four principal considerations relating to the ecology of herbicide use: (1) chemical stability, (2) possible movement of the herbicide from the area of application, (3) bioconcentration effect if any (example: DDT in fish), and (4) the spectrum and degree of toxicity to animals and man, usually referred to as mammalian toxicity, and to aquatic organisms. With some early understanding of physical, chemical and biological phenomena, a great deal of intelligent prediction can be made as to potential hazards. The great variety of herbicides now federally registered and commercially available present the consumer with a remarkably specific arsenal against weeds. A brief description of the very important herbicide atrazine will demonstrate this.

Atrazine, manufactured by Geigy, is one of the most popular herbicides for corn (Figure 1). Effective on many broadleaf and some grassy weeds, it is comparatively stable chemically and may require some 12 to 18 months to dissipate from soils. Atrazine breaks down through microbiological action more rapidly in warm, moist, high-organic soils. The rapidity of breakdown of herbicides, or of any

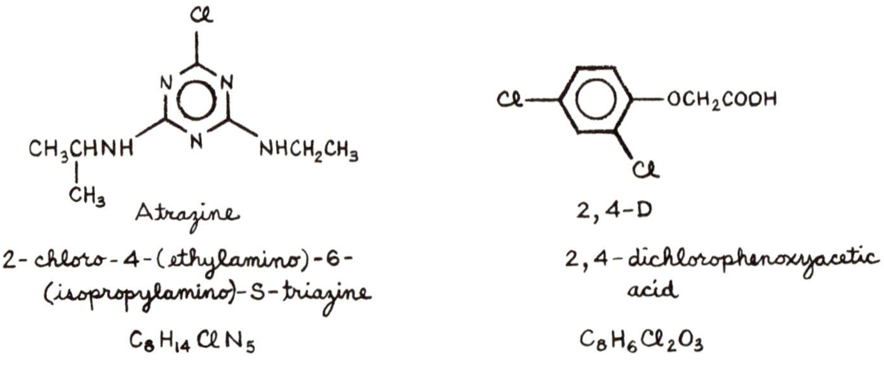

Atrazine

2-chloro-4-(ethylamino)-6-
(isopropylamino)-S-triazine

$C_8H_{14}ClN_5$

2,4-D

2,4-dichlorophenoxyacetic
acid

$C_8H_6Cl_2O_3$

Figure 1: Atrazine and 2,4-D.

organic chemical in the soil for that matter, is a function of temperature, organic matter, and moisture. In dry or low-organic soil, or in cold soils, microbiological degradation rates usually are slow. Because atrazine may persist 12 to 18 months at commonly used application rates there may be risk of injury if sensitive crops (such as soybeans) are planted where atrazine was used the prior year. Where corn follows corn, atrazine may be used safely. It does not move significantly out of the zone of application. It does not show evidence of bioconcentration, and mammalian toxicity is low. Other triazine herbicides are registered for corn and other crops.

Atrazine is a pre-emergence herbicide. The older phenoxy products are used primarily postemergence due to their efficient uptake by weed foliage and the subsequent killing action. Probably the best known and most widely used herbicide 2,4-D (Figure 1) is of this kind. Even though it was discovered some 25 years ago, and has been used extensively for nearly as long, its exact biological action is not yet fully understood. We do know that 2,4-D affects plant respiration, food reserves, and cell function. In general, it selectively controls broadleaf weeds in grass type crops such as turf, pastures, wheat, barley, corn, sorghum, sugarcane, and rice. 2,4-D degrades readily in soil and does not concentrate. The one important problem relative to its use is occasional injury to susceptible crops from physical drift of spray usually caused by wind or by application error. U. S. production of 2,4-D in 1958 approximated 31 million pounds, and this increased to about 79 million pounds ten years later.

THE 2,4,5-T CONTROVERSY

A close relative of 2,4-D is 2,4,5-T (Figure 2). This herbicide is used very effectively for controlling unwanted woody species on

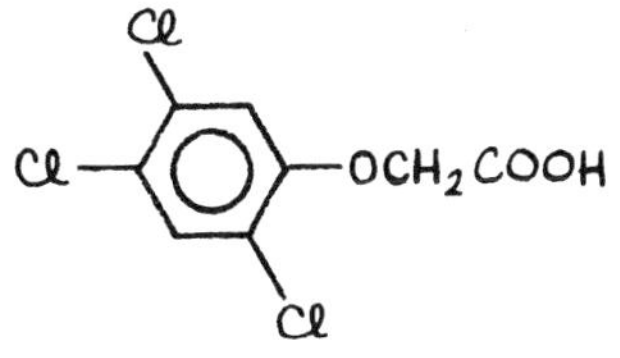

2,4,5-T

2,4,5 - trichlorophenoxyacetic -
acid $C_8H_5Cl_3O_3$

Figure 2: 2,4,5-T.

rangelands and along rights-of-way. It also is used to kill weeds in certain crops such as rice and weed trees in conifer plantings. It is a safe herbicide from the standpoint of mammalian toxicity and it does not persist for long periods in soil. This very useful herbicide has come into prominence recently because of defoliation by the military in Southeast Asia. Originally, the idea was to open up the enemy supply trails and to prevent ambush of allied troops. A mixture of 2,4-D and 2,4,5-T butyl ester was an agent called "orange." The current 2,4, 5-T controversy is an interesting case that touches on public policy, on chemistry, and on the professional responsibilities of chemists and scientists. Here is a brief history of what happened.

At the time this controversy erupted I was serving on the Mrak Commission, appointed by Secretary Finch to investigate the overall environmental and health aspects of pesticide use. This commission was appointed after the discovery of concentrations of DDT in coho salmon in Lake Michigan. One week before the last meeting, October 29, 1969, Dr. Lee Dubridge, Head of the Office of Science and Technology, announced the finding, that 2,4,5-T had caused birth anomalies in experiments sponsored by the National Cancer Institute and conducted by the Bionetics Laboratory. Although the samples had been collected in 1963, and the first tests run in 1964, this report did not reach the public until October, 1969. Up to that time, my membership on the commission had not been complicated by issues surrounding products made by Dow; hence there was no conflict of interest. However, because of the widespread public concern over 2,4,5-T, I thought it best to tender my resignation. I did, but it was not accepted.

In the last meeting I proceeded to question whether or not the sample (produced by a company which no longer makes 2,4,5-T) employed in the NCI test was a truly representative sample. I raised this question because of experience in 1964 when Dow was asked by the Department of Defense to produce quantities of 2,4,5-T beyond the usual capacity of our plant. We raised the temperatures in the reactor to increase the rate of hydrolysis of 1,2,4,5-tetrachlorobenzene to sodium 2,4,5-trichlorophenate, and soon encountered a problem formerly experienced in the days of manufacture of chlorinated phenols. Some of the workers developed a condition known as chlorance. This begins as a pimplelike reddening of the skin followed by acne and blackhead formation. It is slow to heal. This condition had been observed while making trichlorophenol in the 1940's.

A rabbit-ear test had been perfected by V. K. Rowe and E. M. Adams in our Biochemical Research Laboratory, so we could check whether or not the product or the environment, which we sampled by wipe test, were contaminated with an acnegen. The rabbit-ear test was our standard method of monitoring in the 1940's and 1950's. Ten days were required for this test; thus this bioassay was slow to yield readings for industrial hygiene purposes. When we encountered difficulties in 1964, a chromatographic method was developed to monitor the contaminant, then known to be 2,3,7,8-tetrachlorodibenzo-p-dioxin (TCDD). Contaminated 2,4,5-T was not sold by Dow. Rather, we shut down the plant and purchased our supplies of 2,4,5-T from another manufacturer that was not having difficulties. We reported our findings to other manufacturers, redesigned our plant and resumed production in 1966, supplying material which contained no more than 1 part per million of TCDD.

It is important at this point to make a distinction in the processes for making dichlorophenol and trichlorophenol. Dichlorophenol (an intermediate for 2,4-D), is produced by chlorinating phenol itself. But, in the case of trichlorophenol, tetrachlorobenzene is hydrolyzed (Figure 3). In the presence of sodium hydroxide and methanol, sodium 2,4,5-trichlorophenate salt forms. Under more strenuous reaction conditions, such as temperatures above 160°C, two molecules of sodium trichlorophenate will condense to form 2,3,7,8-tetrachlorodibenzo-p-dioxin as a contaminant. This material had been proved to be the cause of chloracne and was known to be toxic. These facts were established by Dow investigators in 1964 and 1965.

This information was reported to the Mrak Commission in early November of 1969. It was suggested that the sample obtained by the NCI and tested by the Bionetics Laboratory may have been contaminated.

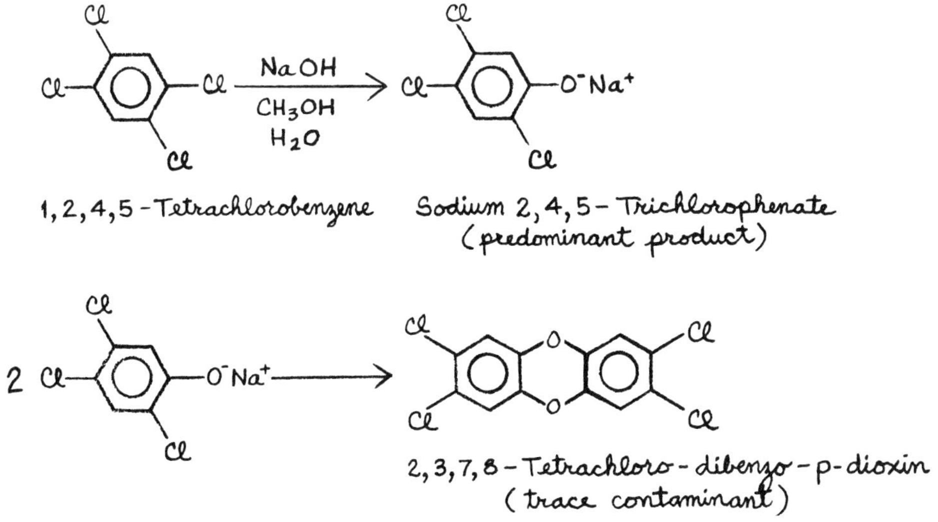

1,2,4,5-Tetrachlorobenzene   Sodium 2,4,5-Trichlorophenate
                                    (predominant product)

2,3,7,8-Tetrachloro-dibenzo-p-dioxin
(trace contaminant)

Figure 3: Formation of 2,3,7,8-tetrachloro-dibenzo-p-dioxin.

Arrangements were made to obtain the original sample for analysis. Experiments were jointly planned, between Dow investigators and representatives of HEW, to retest 2,4,5-T samples of recent manufacture which had contained less than 1 part per million of the suspected tetradioxin.

We conducted the analyses and the Food and Drug Administration confirmed the results. The sample used by the Bionetics Laboratory which caused the birth defects in rats and mice contained 27 ⋅ 8 ppm of 2,3,7,8-tetrachlorodibenzo-p-dioxin. Thus, the crucial sample in question was impure. Since that time, there have been continuing efforts to determine whether or not the so-called teratology effects that were observed were a result of the contaminant or whether 2,4,5-trichlorophenoxyacetic acid itself is teratogenic. Experiments in rats and rabbits (by methods agreed to by all parties concerned) have not produced birth anomalies with commercial 2,4,5-T containing less than 1 ppm 2,3,7,8-tetrachlorodibenzo-p-dioxin. However, in the case of susceptible mice (highly inbred mice which are susceptible to cleft palate) there is a controversy because several investigators claim that 2,4,5-trichlorophenoxy acetic acid causes a significant increase in number of cleft palates when using extremely large dosages of test material which contains 0.1 to 0.2 ppm TCDD. These tests are being repeated, and the controversy continues.

The issue reaches far beyond the importance of 2,4,5-T itself, and involves the adequacy of the original test procedures, the selection of test samples, and the scientific criteria from which public policy is being generated. At the present time, Mr. Ruckelshaus of the Environmental Protection Agency is considering two reports: The Presidential Science Advisory Report on 2,4,5-T, and the Wilson Report, which has been rather recently published. The Wilson Report claims that the ban on 2,4,5-T should essentially be lifted, with the proviso that the specification on the contaminant TCDD be less than 0.1 ppm. The President's Science Advisory Report, published at an earlier date in the absence of recently developed information, states that consumer's caution is indicated.

I want to describe briefly the adequacy of test methods, because that is where the whole issue hinges. On the basis of toxicity alone, we decided to consider unusable any contamination above 1 ppm of 2,4,5-T with 2,3,7,8-tetrachlorodibenzo-p-dioxin. With a specification that TCDD not exceed 0.1 ppm, and with the usages now recommended, there is a wide margin of safety in the use of 2,4,5-T. But, let me get back to some of the questions of teratology as a decisive test method. How valid are the procedures? I would like to paraphrase Dr. Leon Golberg, a well-known toxicologist, who has made a serious study of present methods employed to sustain policy decisions.

"In checking on potential teratogenicity of trace chemical contaminants in food, the height of absurdity is achieved by the combination of a maximum tolerated dose, a parenteral route of administration, and the application of zero tolerance on the basis of results. In this area we know full well that any one of a host of adverse influences on the mother is reflected in fetal deaths, resorptions and/or abnormalities. Teratogenic effects are elicited by: transport of mice by air on days 12 and 13 of pregnancy; fasting for 24 hours or less at a critical stage of gestation, which may be brought about inadvertently or unsuspectingly by inducing somnolence, lethargy, muscle weakness or ataxia; a diet of raisins for one day; severe limitation of movement or avoidance behavior; and many other nonspecific factors probably acting through a stress mechanism, as well as hyper- or hypothermia and endocrine influence. Even subcutaneous sodium chloride is teratogenic in mice. Here, above all, is a situation that demands the utmost care in selecting doses that do not render the mother sufficiently ill to produce even transient inappetance. The use of a maximum tolerated dose overlooks the possibility of non-specific toxic stress . . . ."

This is one of the real issues which faces the government and industry today in the shaping of public policy; to develop a reliable and trustworthy methodology for evaluating risk. Today there is a great deal of concern and public fear about birth defects, mutagens, and carcinogens. I think what we have to strive for is a greater understanding of test methods that can be reliably used so that the public can be reassured and so that industry knows better what is required.

In the case of the particular dioxin associated with some samples of 2,4,5-T, we know that it is degraded in soil, although slowly; it is not mobile; it does not leach. It is not formed from 2,4,5-T in the presence of sunlight, or by burning contaminated foliage.

Eagles which have been sent in to the Department of the Interior for analysis showed detectable concentrations of DDT and polychlorinated biphenyls but no detectable (>0.5 ppm) levels of chlorodioxins.

Experiments run in Dow laboratories with radioactively labelled TCDD in rats showed that about 53 per cent was found in the feces (this is at a 21-day interval), 13.4 per cent was in the urine, and about 3.2 per cent was in the expired air. There was a rapid decline in liver concentration and a reasonably rapid elimination from fat. TCDD does not appear to have the bioconcentration potential that DDT has.

I should mention the toxicity of other dioxins. Dichlorodibenzo-p-dioxin forms with great difficulty and is not present in detectable levels (less than 0.1 ppm) in 2,4-dichlorophenol. Moreover, this dioxin from 2,4-dichlorophenol is not highly toxic. Hence any dioxin problem in connection with 2,4-D is remote and of no consequence. Sodium penta-chlorophenate under certain conditions will convert to small amounts of the octachlorodibenzo-p-dioxin. Tests of 90 days' duration in rats have indicated a low order of toxicity for this compound. The toxicities in decreasing order are tetra> hexa> hepta> di> octa-chlorodibenzo-p-dioxin.

GENERATING PUBLIC POLICY

In conclusion, I would like to make a few suggestions for the future in regard to the generation of public policy.

In the first place, the government should do a better job of defining test requirements. The test methods of protocols, however, need flexibility for individual judgment, *and* provision for deliberate change. Change in requirements should not be capricious but should derive from advances in science and advances in knowledge. Any change, however, should involve understanding and participation by industry, not by sudden unilateral government decree. Changes should be made with good and sufficient reason based on facts.

Another suggestion is that a mechanism be developed for certification of toxicological laboratories. This means industrial, university, commercial, and government laboratories. Greater public confidence could be developed for the results issuing from such laboratories if certification required that a qualifying board periodically rule on the adequacy of personnel, procedures, equipment, and housing. The objective should be to improve and make more uniform the quality of the data used for support of consumer products.

Assuming that laboratories could be certified, then only toxicological data from certified laboratories should be admissible for the support of product registration or for the support of residue tolerance. It is further suggested that the second supplier of a pesticide, after the original petitioner's patent expires, be permitted to purchase certified data. This could be purchased either from the original supplier or perhaps from a government agency. The main objective would be to burden the second supplier so that he does not have an unfair competitive advantage compared to the one who has borne the original cost of development.

With a provision of certified data being the only type of toxicological data admissible for support of tolerance, and with the requirement that the second supplier be required to pay his way, it would be possible to lay the registration and the tolerance petitions open for inspection and to encourage publication. Openness of the data at this point would satisfy many objections. Today neither the qualified investigator nor the public has access to the facts; hence the public is suspicious. The experiment stations, expected to help support the use of a product, do not have access to certain registration information. Experiment stations and extension specialists need confidence in the validity of the backup information. Furthermore, the public official charged with registration and tolerance proceedings is under pressure because the present policy forbids him from making certain information available without consent of the petitioner. The whole situation promotes public distrust because supporting facts are not out in the open.

EQUITABLE REGULATIONS

We should more aggressively extend the use of the experimental label prior to full registration so that typical though limited sale can be achieved under qualified supervision. This would permit the development of meaningful use experience with limited exposure of the total population. The objective would be to discover unexpected phenomena difficult or impossible to elucidate under laboratory or limited field test conditions.

One of the weakest links in the chain is in diagnosis of pest problems and application of pesticides. I do not wish to discredit those competent professionals who do a good job. Nevertheless, in the country at large, the process of diagnosis and application involves people who are often unskilled, poorly paid, and nonprofessional. We have many elegant tools but poor craftsmen. To overcome this difficulty, I would suggest that we classify pesticides in two categories—for professional use only, and for nonprofessional use. Those for professional use could be applied by licensed professionals only, people skilled in diagnosis and application. As there is a scarcity of this kind of skill, training of a new kind of professional should be developed by our agricultural schools. This will take time, but it is needed and the professional licenses should be granted only to those qualified. The grower would then pay for results and the whole process of pest control, including weed control, would be less poundage oriented and more result oriented. This will require some rethinking on the part of industry as to how they can make their contribution and reap their share of the reward.

There is economic room to maneuver if everyone is compelled to compete by equitable regulations. The whole cost structure will be elevated, to be sure, and these costs will be borne by the ultimate consumer.

I think we need a new sensitivity in this whole area of professional responsibility, and to you who are chemists or chemists-in-the-making, I cannot overemphasize how dependent we in industry or in government are on the credibility and trustworthiness of the data that you create in the laboratory. Much unnecessary public fear and consternation are being generated by the dissemination of half-baked results, inadequate experiments, improperly-designed tests, which have not been reviewed by peer groups capable of review—where the investigator has succumbed to the temptation to get his name in the paper!

Science, in my opinion, has lost some of its allure in the public mind. I think one of the things that we must do as scientists is to improve our credibility. We must generate trustworthy information and explain our stand in a more articulate manner to the public at large.

Senator Ribicoff conducted hearings on the pesticide issue in 1963. A report of hearings published in 1966 contains the following passage.

THE RESPONSIBILITIES OF THE SCIENTIST

The committee asked the scientific witnesses for meaningful advice for the Congress, but much of the testimony was inhibited by defense of past positions, employer loyalties, and lack of authority.

Scientists should do as thorough a job of preparing answers on aspects of research administration and planning as they do on the technical details of the work.

The maker of public policy must have alternatives from which to choose. There are always strong vested interests which resist change. Unless the technological situation (in this case, ecology) can be clearly explained and related to public policy issues, the decision-maker is hard put to recommend any new course. This understanding must be extended also to the citizen. No great social issues have ever been decided until the needs were clear to the man in the street.

Scientists cannot assume that their knowledge will reach the decision-maker through the normal channels of publication and review in the scientific community. Without shortcutting the classical methods of assessing the truth, there is still an obligation to interpret what is known and replace emotion, rumor, and misconception with a clear explanation of the facts.

The role of the scientist in relation to the legislator is limited to an area somewhere short of the decision-making point. Proper use of scientific advice requires considerable effort on both the part of the scientific community and the body politic.

SUGGESTED READING

Kearney, P. C. and D. D. Kaufman, Degradation of Herbicides, New York, Marcel Dekker, Inc., 1969.

Klingman, Glenn C., Weed Control As A Science, New York, John Wiley and Sons, Inc., 1961.

PESTS AND POLLUTION

Challenge of Modern Insect Control

Robert L. Metcalf

DDT is an acronym for the chemical insecticide dichlorodiphenyl-trichloroethane, a compound which probably has had more influence upon the human race than any other substance yet invented.

Man has long sought practical means for protecting himself, his domestic animals, and his food supply from the attacks of thousands of species of noxious insects. The damage that such insects cause is enormously magnified by the activities of certain biting species in transmitting diseases between animal reservoirs and man. Plague is caused by *Pasteurella pestis*, and spread from rats to man by the bites of the Oriental rat flea *Xenopsylla cheopis* and other fleas. Plague is estimated to have killed 100 million people during the first great plague of the Sixth Century and another 25 million during a second plague of the Fourteenth Century. Plague in India caused almost 19 million deaths from 1896 to 1917. The disease is still a threat to world health. Epidemic typhus is caused by *Rickettsia prowazekii* and is transmitted to man by the human body louse *Pediculus humanus*. Typhus caused the death of more than 2.5 millions of Russians during the First World War. Millions more died in the Balkans, Poland, and Germany. African sleeping sickness, caused by the protozoan *Trypansoma gambiense* and *T. rhodiense*, and transmitted by the tsetse flies *Glossina* spp., caused about 500 thousand deaths from 1896 to 1906. The ravages of the tsetse fly in spreading sleeping sickness, and the closely related cattle disease, nagana, have prevented the modern economic development of about 4.5 million square miles of Africa.

Malaria, a protozoan disease caused by *Plasmodia* and transmitted by the bites of more than 85 species of *Anopheles* mosquitoes, has long been the most important human disease. Before the advent of DDT, malaria caused approximately 200 million clinical cases and 2.5 million deaths. As late as 1958, an epidemic in Ethiopia resulted in 3 million victims, of which 100,000 died. In 1968 Ceylon suffered a malaria epidemic of more than 1 million cases.

DDT has been used since 1939 to control the insect vectors of these and other human diseases. Dr. Edward Knipling estimated in 1943 that the chemical had probably saved over 5 million lives, and prevented some 100 million illnesses. The reckoning by 1971 must be at least 10 times as impressive, because of the much wider scope of utilization of DDT, especially in the World Health Organization Programme for the Eradication of Malaria.

HISTORY OF DDT

The original synthesis of DDT was made by a German doctoral student, Othmar Zeidler, who was working in the laboratory of Adolph von Baeyer at the University of Strasburg. In 1873 Zeidler was studying the condensation of chloral, a hypnotic drug, with various substituted benzenes in the presence of sulfuric acid. This reaction has subsequently become known as the Baeyer Condensation. On one occasion, Zeidler used chlorobenzene and condensed two moles of this substance with one mole of chloral to produce 2,2-bis- (p-chlorophenyl)-1,1,1-trichloroethane, or DDT.

chlorobenzene   chloral   DDT-carbinol   DDT

It is interesting to speculate what might have happened if a stray cockroach or housefly had blundered into the pile of shining needlelike crystals of DDT (mp 110°C) as they lay drying on Zeidler's laboratory bench. Would the insect's dying struggles have caught the discoverer's attention, and would he have traced the cause to DDT? Alas, the good fairy Serendipity was elsewhere, and the miraculous power of DDT was to remain undiscovered for another 65 years. Othmar Zeidler's inaugural dissertation "Uber Verbindungen von chloral mit Brom- und Chlorbenzol" was published in 1874. He went on to a postdoctoral appointment in Lieben's laboratory in Vienna and published moderately from 1875 to 1879 and then his name seems to have disappeared from the chemical literature.

Zeidler's mentor, Adolph von Baeyer, was a man of profound influence on the profession of chemistry. He gave the inaugural address of the Deutschen Chemischen Gesellschaft in 1868 and was perhaps the most illustrious German chemist of the era. At the age of 80 he still lectured and directed classes. One feels that Baeyer, the 1905 Nobel Laureate in chemistry "in recognition of his services in the development of organic chemistry and the chemical industry through his work on organic dyes and hydroaromatic combinations," would have thoroughly enjoyed the practical discovery of the insecticide DDT.

The discovery of the insecticidal properties of DDT occurred in the laboratories of the company J. R. Geigy, A. G., a venerable Swiss dyestuff manufacturer. Geigy had been interested in the development of mothproofing agents for a number of years. One of their products, Mitin FF, described as a colorless dyestuff which could be firmly fixed to wool by the interaction of its sulfonic acid moiety, was employed during the dyeing process to protect woolen fabrics permanently against clothes moths and carpet beetles.

Mitin FF

Mitin FF contains the p,p-dichlorodiphenylether moiety which Geigy scientists considered to be the portion of the molecule responsible for mothproofing qualities (toxiphore). Dr. Paul Muller was seeking simpler lipidsoluble compounds which would be effective as contact insecticides. During his methodical investigation of compounds containing the bis- (p-chlorophenyl) moiety, he repeated Zeidler's synthesis and, on September 25, 1939, found that DDT was extraordinarily effective against fabric pests and a variety of other insects as well. The extent of Paul Muller's success is measured by the award of the 1948

Nobel Prize in Physiology and Medicine "for your discovery of the strong action of DDT against a wide variety of arthropods."

DDT was born in a world just plunged into the catastrophy of World War II. Military hygientists had vivid memories of the ravages of louse-borne typhus, which in World War I was a critical factor in the collapse of the Balkans and in the defeat of Russian armies on the Eastern Front. Moreover, the rapid extension of hostilities to North Africa, and later to the South Pacific, brought the mosquito-transmitted diseases of malaria, filariasis, and dengue fever into sharp focus as important military elements in victory and defeat. Both sides of the conflict were engaged in research on an unprecedented scale to find better chemical weapons to control these insect vectors of disease. The neutral Swiss were in a strategic position to exploit their extraordinary discovery. During the next several years, both tales of the insecticidal potency of DDT and samples of technical DDT, a greasy white powder with a faint smell of ripe apples, found their way to research centers in Europe and the United States.

Entomologists were generally skeptical. After all, the best weapons available to combat lice and mosquitoes were the very expensive and short-lived pyrethrins; it seemed unlikely that a new synthetic substance could be even more toxic to insects, last for months on treated surfaces, and be so safe that humans and animals could be liberally dusted or sprayed without any ill effects. That all this could be achieved in a simple chemical costing only about 1/100 as much as the pyrethrins boggled the imagination. Extensive tests by the Orlando, Florida laboratory of the U.S. Department of Agriculture confirmed all the original claims and extended the areas of usefulness manyfold. DDT rapidly became the chief weapon for the control of insects of military importance, and played a major role in protecting U.S. troops against malaria and other mosquito-borne diseases in the South Pacific, and against typhus in North Africa and Europe. Thus was the age of its exploitation begun.

DDT AS AN INSECTICIDE

DDT is in many ways the perfect insecticide. A white crystalline powder with a faint fruity odor, it is effective against almost all insects, posseses extreme durability and persistence, exhibits low toxic hazard to man and higher animals, and is available at low cost (18.5¢ per lb in 1970). DDT is a highly selective insecticide: it is very readily absorbed by the lipoprotein cuticle of insects, but not by the mammalian skin. As an example, the American cockroach *Periplaneta* is killed by application to the body of doses of 10 mg per kg of body weight; when injected intraperitoneally, the lethal dose is only reduced to 8 mg per kg. In the rat a much greater resistance to contact is seen. Doses of 3000 mg per kg of body weight are required for death on contact, while only 150 mg per kg is fatal when injected intraperitoneally. An even smaller dose of 50 mg per kg is lethal when injected into the bloodstream.

The use of DDT reached a peak of 800 million pounds per year in 1961, with U.S. production at about 160 million pounds. A total of more than 4 billion pounds has been used for insect control since 1940, of which about four-fifths has gone to control pests of agriculture and forestry, and the remainder has been used in public health. World production remains greater than 400 million pounds per year. At the height of its use (1961), DDT was registered for use on 334 agricultural commodities.

DDT gave phenomenal results compared to the arsenical insecticides, which it replaced. The average potato yield in New York State in the period 1936 to 1945, under the best growing practices and treatment with lead arsenate, was 110 bushels per acre. In 1946 and 1947, the first years that DDT was used extensively to control potato pests, the average yield was 172 bushels per acre, a 56 per cent increase. When applied to apples and other deciduous fruits, DDT gave exceptional control of the codling moth and other pests. The damage to apples in Illinois orchards in 1956 to 1958 averaged only 2.2 per cent as compared to 69 per cent in unsprayed trees. DDT was exceptionally effective against the two great defoliators of American forest trees: the gypsy moth in the East, and the spruce budworm in the West. Hundreds of thousands of acres were sprayed by air. DDT became the principal cotton insecticide, especially effective against bollworm and pink bollworm. The agent was very widely used to control the ravages of the elm-bark beetles that spread the deadly Dutch Elm disease. DDT became a household word as a most effective mothproofing remedy against clothes moths and carpet beetles. There is no doubt that DDT has contributed immensely to food and fiber production throughout the world.

The safety record of DDT in pest control is extraordinary. Whole populations have had 10 per cent DDT powder blown into their clothing as they wore it to control human body lice and prevent typhus. In areas undergoing eradication of malaria, millions of humans have lived for nearly a generation in homes where interior walls and ceilings have been sprayed with DDT at 1 g per m^2 every year (this practice is referred to as residual spraying). Most plants and animals eaten by man have been treated with DDT and contain trace residues of this substance.

Despite this ubiquitous and persistent use of DDT, and the heavy occupational exposure of thousands who manufacture, formulate, and spray DDT, there is no authenticated case of death resulting from exposure to DDT. The only human illnesses attributed to it are those resulting from massive ingestion either by accident or through suicidal intent.

DDT IN TYPHUS CONTROL

Typhus has always existed in epidemic proportions during the filth and misery of wartime. A 5 per cent DDT louse powder was evaluated in 1942 and proposed for the control of typhus. Techniques for the mass delousing of humans without removal of clothing were developed by the Rockefeller Foundation Typhus Team in Algiers in 1943. These procedures were given a severe trial in a typhus epidemic in Naples in July 1943. During a seven-month period more than 3,265,786 individual applications of DDT powder were made. The epidemic ended with only 1403 cases of typhus.

Typhus became established in Germany shortly after the beginning of World War II and was especially severe in the Dachau and Belsen concentration camps. In the Belsen camp there were estimated to be more than 20,000 cases from January to April 1945, when the camp was liberated by the British. At this time all 61,000 inmates were universally infested by lice and there were 3,500 cases of typhus. All inmates were dusted with DDT by the ninth day after liberation; the onset of typhus ceased by the fourteenth day. Only 3 per cent of the inhabitants had lice at the conclusion of the treatments. It is difficult to overestimate the role of DDT in preventing major epidemics of typhus throughout Europe following the release of these inmates of concentration camps. Stanhope Bayne-Jones summed it up: "The Conclusion is warranted that for the first time in the history of typhus in wartime, epidemics of the disease were brought under control before they had run their previously customary course."

DDT IN MALARIA CONTROL

The most impressive use of DDT has been in residual house spraying for malaria control. Previous to the development of DDT, effective control of this disease was feasible only in very limited geographic areas where mosquito control could be economically effected by drainage, house screening, space spraying, and various techniques of killing larvae. It was discovered during World War II that DDT applied to the interior surfaces of dwellings at 1 to 2 g per m^2 would remain insecticidal to adult anopheline mosquitoes for six months to one year. The adult female anopheline mosquito vectors of malaria habitually invade human habitations for a nocturnal blood meal about every two days. However, since 10 to 20 days are required for the ingested gametocytes of *Plasmodium* to produce infective sporozoites in the salivary glands of the mosquito, and as the latter doubles her body weight during the blood meal, the chances of her resting on a DDT-treated surface are very great if all habitations are routinely sprayed. Thus, the transmission of malaria is interrupted at a 'weak point' between the formation of gametocytes and sporozoites. This simple public health measure was applied by the Italian entomologist A. Missiroli to the Latina province of Italy, a potentially rich agricultural area which had suffered from endemic malaria since the beginning of recorded history. Spraying was begun in the area of the Pontine marshes on June 5, 1945. After two years of spraying all dwellings with 5 per cent DDT in kerosene at about 2 g per m^2 of surface the vectors *Anopheles labranchiae* and *A. sacharovi* had virtually disappeared. The number of cases of malaria declined, and by midsummer of 1949 no more cases of malaria were recorded.

At about the same time the International Health Division of the Rockefeller Foundation inaugurated a demonstration in malaria eradication on the island of Sardinia. Under the direction of John Logan, a dynamic sanitary engineer, all the dwellings and other adult resting sites, together with larval breeding areas, were treated with DDT beginning on October 1, 1945. The results demonstrated the astounding efficiency of DDT (Table 1). There has been no evidence of the

TABLE 1
Elimination of Malaria from Sardinia by DDT Treatment.

Year	Total Cases of Malaria
1944	78,173
1945	74,641
1946	75,447
1947	39,303
1948	15,121
1949	1,314
1950	44
1951	9

transmission of malaria after 1950. The disappearance of the disease brought about great economic changes in an island which, as recently as 1950, was described as a "mountainous, unhealthy, infertile region." Sardinia has now become a new playground in the Mediterranean, and has changed from a goat- and sheep-herding economy to a grain-growing agriculture and is a prosperous industrial region.

An unexpected finding in the Sardinian experiment was that the vector A. *labranchiae,* which declined to a very low population level, was not eradicated. This program gave rise to the new concept of "anophelism without malaria" and set the stage for the World Health Organization Programme for the worldwide eradication of malaria.

Worldwide Malaria Eradication

From the early spectacular successes it was clear that malaria could be brought under complete control by residual house spraying, at a cost much lower than the relatively expensive programs which involved drainage of swamps and destruction of larvae. By 1950 nearly all of the North and South American countries with malaria problems were engaged in serious efforts of control by DDT sprays. In that year the Pan-American Sanitary Bureau recommended that a coordinated plan be devised to achieve continental eradication of malaria. The development of serious DDT resistance in the housefly and in *Anopheles sacharovi* in Greece in 1949 added impetus to planning.

In May 1955 the Joint Health Committee of UNICEF/WHO recommended the eradication of malaria. Simultaneously, the World Health Assembly proposed that WHO should "take the initiative, provide the technical advice, and encourage research and coordination of resources in the implementation of a programme having as its ultimate objective the worldwide eradication of Malaria." Thus began what is probably the largest biological experiment of all time. As of 1971 the use of persistent pesticides, notably DDT, protects 1,329 million people, out of a total of 1,802 million, living in originally malarious areas of 146 countries. Malaria has been pronounced as eradicated in 36 countries, either highly developed or islands, with a total population of 710 million. An additional 27 countries have large-scale programs, and another 53 have programs in various stages of success. Thirty countries, mostly in Africa, with more than 360 million inhabitants, have no projects for eradication.

The immediate results of the eradication of malaria have astonished even the visionaries. In India, DDT-residual spraying decreased the cases of malaria from 100 million annually, in the period 1933 to

1935, to 150,000 by 1966, with a consequent decrease in deaths from 750,000 to 1,500. In Ceylon, after a country-wide DDT spraying campaign, the number of malaria cases fell from 2.8 million in 1946 to 17 in 1963; deaths fell from 12,587 to zero. In this period the general death rate fell from 20.3 to 8.6 per thousand, and infant mortality from 141 to 57 per thousand. The use of DDT has provided death control on an unprecedented scale. In addition, DDT has proven a major factor in increasing longevity. The length of life in India rose from about 32 years in 1948 to 52 years in 1970. Thus, the use of DDT is an important contributing factor to the population explosion.

The economic benefits from malaria control programs are easy to demonstrate. DDT residual house spraying costs from 11¢ to 44¢ per capita per year, in various parts of the world. WHO has calculated that malaria in India cost the economy $1,300 million in 1935; this has now been reduced to $2 million annually, with a total expenditure for control of only $200 million. The dramatic effects of DDT-residual spraying on the malaria-mosquito-man ecosystem are nowhere better illustrated than by recent experiences in Ceylon. In this country 66,704 people died of malaria in 1934 and 1935; there were 2.8 million cases of malaria in 1946. As shown in Table 2, DDT residual spraying rapidly decreased the incidence of malaria to almost zero in 1963. Spraying was prematurely terminated in 1964 without achieving eradication and its cessation was followed by a violent epidemic of more than 2.5 million cases in 1968 and 1969.

TABLE 2
Recrudescence of Malaria in Ceylon Following Termination of DDT Spraying (data from WHO)

Year		Total cases of malaria
1946		2,800,000
1962		32
1963		17
1964	(spraying terminated)	150
1965		308
1966		499
1967		3,466
1968	January 16,493	> 1,000,000
	February 42,161	

DDT AND THE ENVIRONMENT

The other side of the coin is the role of DDT as an environmental micropollutant. DDT is the classic example of these substances because of its extreme insolubility in water (to about 0.002 ppm) and its high lipid solubility (to about 100,000 ppm). Thus DDT has a partition coefficient in lipid/water approaching infinity. The same is true of its principal degradation product, DDE, whose properties are very similar. Worse yet, DDE is even more stable. DDT and DDE may persist in soils for 10 years or more and can be redistributed by erosion. It is estimated that of the more than 4 billion pounds of DDT which have been liberated into the environment, as much as 25 per cent of this total is in circulation in the global ecosystem either as DDT or DDE. Thus it is not surprising that human beings from ten countries have averages of 4.3 ppm DDT and 4.8 ppm of DDE in their body fat, with extremes ranging from 0.8 ppm DDT and 2.2 ppm DDE in Alaskan Eskimos, to 648 ppm DDT and 483 ppm DDE in a worker in a DDT factory. These concentrations in storage in the human body have produced no observable ill effects, but are clearly undesirable. The DDT in storage is slowly metabolized (it has a biological half life of about 6 months) by the scheme shown in Figure 1. After metabolism, the initial DDT is excreted in urine as DDA. This mechanism causes an eventual steady-state or plateau level to be attained in the storage of DDT in laboratory animals and in man. If intake of DDT is prevented, the levels in storage gradually decline.

When fed to animals in trace quantities, DDT is very rapidly stored in the body fat and may be directly absorbed and stored by fish and other aquatic organisms. Fish generally metabolize and excrete DDT at much lower rates than do mammals. In some species of fish, absorption of DDT from water is almost exclusively a product of concentration and length of exposure. Large aging fish may accumulate body burdens ranging from tens to hundreds of ppm of DDT. The processes of body accumulation are further amplified by ecological magnification through food-chain organisms, so that the carnivorous animals at the upper end of the food chain may contain DDT and DDE at levels thousands to millions of times greater than the concentration in water. This is a particularly serious problem in large fresh-water lakes and in estuaries, and is becoming a general phenomenon in the oceans.

The situation in Lake Michigan provides an excellent example. DDT is present in the bottom muds of the lake at concentrations of 14 ppb or more, where it has leached from heavy applications for control of orchard pests and the vector of Dutch Elm disease, the elm-bark beetle. However, the concentration in the water of the lake is only

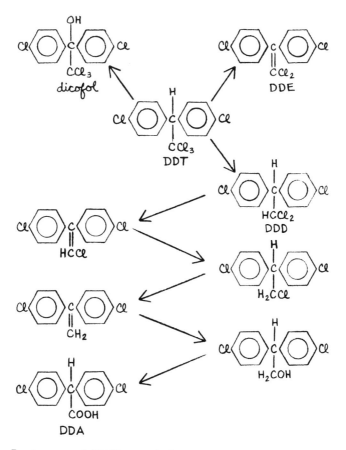

Figure 1: Pathways of DDT metabolism.

about 0.000002 ppm (2 ppt). The amphipods which are an important source of fish food contain about 0.410 ppm (410 ppb), the coho and lake trout 3 to 6 ppm, while the herring gulls feeding on the fish contain 99 ppm. The overall concentration from water to birds is greater than ten million times. Because of the heavy deposits in bottom muds and the very long water retention time in Lake Michigan (30.8 years), pollution by DDT and DDE is virtually irreversible. Many Lake Michigan fish contain levels of DDT in excess of the level of 5 ppm which has been established as safe by the Food and Drug Administration.

Similar problems exist with DDT in the oceans, where DDT has been reported in oysters up to 4.5 ppm, tuna fish to 2 ppm, whales to 6 ppm, and petrels to 10 ppm. The highest concentrations are found in the bodies of fish-eating raptorial birds, such as the peregrine falcon, where amounts of DDE up to 100 ppm have been recorded, with lipid concentrations as high as 5000 ppm of combined DDT and DDE.

Although the exact mechanism of action is in dispute, there is reliable evidence to suggest that levels of DDT and DDE of this magnitude can produce serious reproductive difficulties in a variety of invertebrates, fish, and birds. Both DDT and DDE induce abnormal levels of the multifunction oxidase enzymes in the livers of birds and animals at levels as low as 5 ppm in the diet. These drug-metabolizing enzymes are responsible for converting lipid-soluble xenobiotic compounds into water-soluble and readily-excreted metabolites. The enzymes thus induced may also act on endogenous steroids such as estrogens and androgens, reducing their concentrations. Peakall has shown that pigeons fed DDT have lower estrogen levels than control pigeons, and this mechanism has obvious reproductive consequences. Both DDT and DDE are potent inhibitors of carbonic anhydrase, an enzyme involved in the deposition of calcium carbonate in eggshells. These two biochemical mechanisms offer plausible cause-and-effect relationships between environmental pollution by DDT and DDE and the increasingly visible phenomenon of declining populations of fish-eating birds caused by abnormally thin eggshells which break during incubation.

BIODEGRADABLE AND PERSISTENT ANALOGUES OF DDT

The DDT family is now a large one. Hundreds of related molecules are known that have the proper stereochemical configuration to fit the "DDT—receptor"—that sensitive portion of the nerve axon where DDT interacts. This close molecular absorption results in ion leaks and depolarization of the axon, with the characteristic multiple discharges that produce the tremors and convulsions typical of DDT poisoning. Although 30 years of intensive study have not specifically identified this site, the pronounced similarity of DDT-like action between bioisoteres such as DDT and its totally methylated analogue provides elegant proof of its existence. These two molecules represent the approximate structural limits within which DDT-like action will be found.

2,2-bis (p-chlorophenyl)-   3,3-bis- (p-tolyl)-2,2-dimethylpropane
1,1,1-trichloroethane "DDT"

The use of analogues of DDT for insect control is not new. The bis-p-fluoro analogue "Gix" was used by General Rommel's Afrika Corps for military hygiene in World War II. Methoxychlor, or 2,2-bis-(p-methoxyphenyl) -1,1,1-trichloroethane, was first synthesized by Elbs in 1893; its insecticidal properties were described by Lauger and his colleagues together with those of DDT. However, as it is somewhat less persistent and more expensive than DDT, its usage has been limited, although it is much less acutely toxic to mammals.

2,2-bis-(p-fluorophenyl)-   2,2-bis-(p-methoxyphenyl)-
1,1,1-trichloroethane, "Gix"   1,1,1-trichloroethane, "methoxychlor"

Our laboratory has been interested in studying the biodegradability of DDT and its analogues, with the specific objective of finding persistent yet biodegradable analogues which could substitute for DDT in many environmental uses. Using radiolabeled molecules of DDT and of methoxychlor we investigated the metabolic pathways of the two compounds in insects, mice, and in a "model ecosystem" as shown in Figures 1, 2 and 3. The results were highly productive. In living tissues, as shown in Figure 1, DDT is metabolized partly by dehydrochlorination to DDE—which is very stable and is the important environmental pollutant—and partly by reductive dechlorination to form DDD or 2,2-bis-(p-chlorophenyl) -1,1-dichloroethane. DDD can be further reductively dechlorinated and eventually forms 4,4-dichlorodiphenyl acetic acid, the principal excretory metabolite. All of the intermediate metabolites are strongly lipid partioning and are environmental pollutants.

Methoxychlor, on the other hand, is readily O-demethylated by the mixed function oxidases of the vertebrate liver to form mono- and bisphenols (Figure 2). These are much more water-partioning and can be conjugated and eliminated from the animal body. The comparison of DDT and methoxychlor applied as radiotracers to the Sorghum plants at the terrestrial end of the model ecosystem is particularly informative. After 30 days in this system, large amounts of DDT were recovered together with DDE and DDD. These were concentrated through food

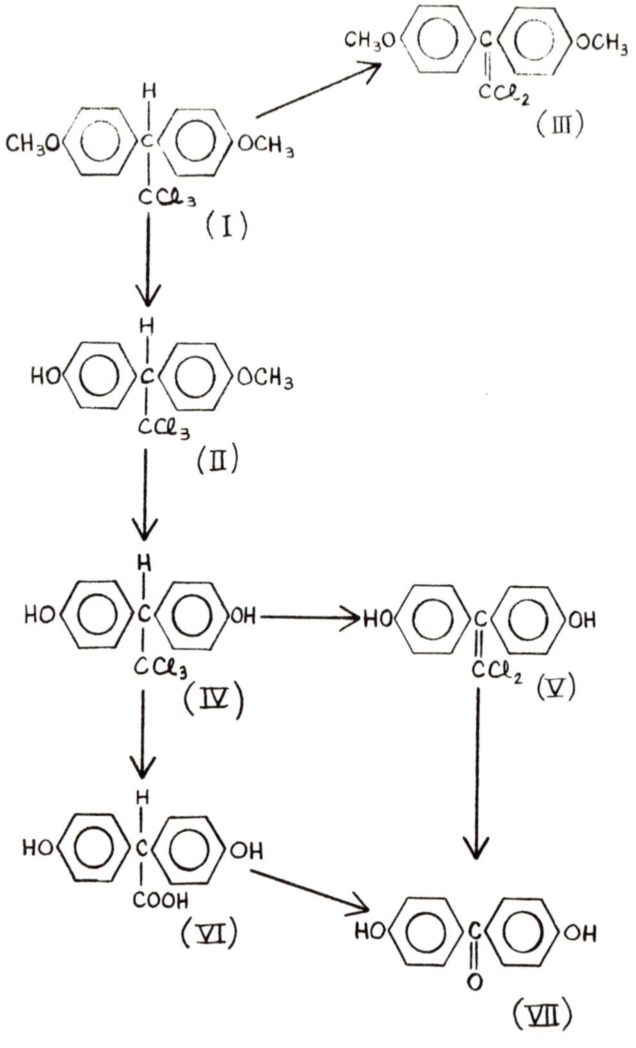

Figure 2: Pathways of methoxychlor metabolism.

chains and stored in the *Gambusia* fish to levels about 50,000 to 100,000 times those in the water. When methoxychlor was applied to the system, it was recovered, as shown in Table 3, largely as the mono- and bis-phenols. The level of concentration in the fish was only about 1000-fold. Additional studies have shown that methoxychlor is rapidly metabolized and eliminated by several species of fish. Methoxychlor is altogether a much more suitable pesticide than DDT for a variety of uses, such as control of blackflies and the bark beetle vectors of Dutch Elm disease.

TABLE 3
**Comparison of the Metabolism of ^{14}C-DDT and ^{3}H-Methoxychlor
in a Model Ecosystem[1]**

	Concentration (ppm)			
	H_2O	Physa (snail)	Culex (mosquito)	Gambusia (fish)
I. DDT				
Total ^{14}C	0.004	22.9	8.9	54.2
DDT	0.00022	7.6	1.8	18.6
DDE	0.00026	12.0	5.2	29.2
DDD	0.00012	1.6	0.4	5.3
polar-metabolites	0.0032	0.98	1.5	0.8
II. Methoxychlor				
Total ^{3}H	0.0016	15.7	0.48	0.33
methoxychlor (I)	0.00011	13.2	-	0.17
methoxychlor ethylene (III)		0.7	-	-
$HOC_6H_4CHCCl_3C_6H_4OCH_3$ (II)	0.00013	1.0	-	-
$HOC_6H_4CCCl_2C_6H_4OH$ (V)	0.00003	-	-	-
polar metabolites	0.00125	0.8	-	0.16
unknown	0.00009	-	-	-

[1]See captions to Figures 1 and 2 for structures associated with names.

These results encouraged us to look at a variety of DDT analogues with substituent groups which could be attacked by the multifunction oxidase of the vertebrate liver, and thus serve as handles for biodegradability. These enzymes can readily attack DDT analogues of three major types to form more polar products as shown below:

We have investigated a considerable number of symmetrical and asymmetrical analogues of DDT containing these biodegradable handles. As shown in Table 4, some of these are highly insecticidal; all are much less acutely toxic to mice than is DDT. They are also biodegradable in model ecosystem evaluations (Figure 3), and do not concentrate

TABLE 4
Toxicity of Some Biodegradable Analogues of DDT to Housefly and Mouse

LD_{50} (mg. per kg.)

R^1	R^2	Housefly - topical	Mouse - oral
Cl	Cl (DDT)	14.0	200
CH_3O	CH_3O (methoxychlor)	45.0	185
C_2H_5O	C_2H_5O	7.0	300-325
CH_3	CH_3	100	3350
CH_3S	CH_3S	225	1000
Cl	CH_3	62.5	-
Cl	CH_3O	41.5	-
CH_3	CH_3O	23.5	>1000
CH_3	C_2H_5O	9.0	1000
CH_3O	CH_3S	32.0	1000

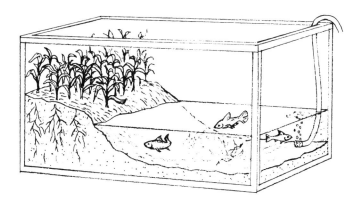

Figure 3: A laboratory model ecosystem with terrestrial-water interface for studying pesticide biogradability and ecological magnification.

appreciably in food chains. We believe there is a considerable future for such persistent, biodegradable, insecticides. They are potentially cheap and could be used to replace DDT in a variety of uses where environmental quality is of paramount concern.

DDT AND HUMAN ECOLOGY

The story of DDT is a perfect illustration of the complexities of human ecology and of the intricate interrelationships that govern the lives and populations of all living organisms. It illustrates the dilemma of our modern industrial society which has with DDT solved enormous problems of public health and food production only to create even more vast problems of environmental pollution and overpopulation.

It is extremely difficult to estimate the risk benefit ratios and the second, third, and further ordered consequences of the use of new discoveries, such as DDT was in 1939. On balance we must conclude that DDT has brought health and contentment to hundreds of millions of people and has saved tens of millions of human lives. It has served not only as the prototype for successful chemical pest control, but also has been an urgently needed indicator of the dangers of indiscriminate environmental pollution. Methoxychlor or other biodegradable analogues of DDT should be substituted for it in all cases where deliberate environmental pollution of soil, fields, forests, lakes, and streams are concerned. However, for essential public health uses in vector control DDT will continue to be a major weapon. The World Health Organization has stated "Indoor spraying with DDT in routine anti-malaria operations does not involve a significant risk to man or wildlife and the withdrawal of this insecticide would be a major tragedy for human health. The outdoor use of DDT is a different matter and effort should be made to avoid it. Biodegradable chemicals should be substituted whenever possible...."

SUGGESTED READINGS

Kapoor, I. P., Metcalf, R. L., Nystrom, R. F., and Sangha, G. K., Comparative metabolism of methoxychlor, methiochlor, and DDT in mouse, insects, and a model ecosystem, *J. Agri. Food Chem.,* 18:1145, 1970.

Levi, G., Sardinia Reborn, *World Health Magazine,* 13:25, 1968.

Metcalf, R. L., Kapoor, I. P., and Hirwe, A., Biodegradable analogues of DDT, *Bull. World Health Org.,* 44:363, 1971.

THE MEAT WE EAT

The Role of Pharmacology in Drug Analysis

William G. Huber

PHARMACOLOGY AND DRUGS

The word pharmacology was originally derived from two Greek words, *pharmacon,* drugs in the mystic sense, and *logos,* a discourse on drugs. Modern pharmacology is defined as the study of the responses of living organisms to drugs. Drugs are chemicals that alter the function or structure of living tissue. Thus the term drug includes far more than is usually the focus of newspaper stories, those mystical drugs that excite or depress the central nervous system.

The drug industry in America is very important, measured either by its contributions to man's welfare or by its dollar volume of business. It is not unusual for the pharmaceutical industry to reckon its annual monetary turnover in billions of dollars. For example, if a company can market a new tranquilizer, the sales potential could be 40 to 50 million dollars per year. If a company successfully markets an antibiotic with desirable features, or a steroid, the current market would be approximately 100 million dollars per year. The drug industry is also vitally involved in areas other than drugs used in man. Herbicides and pesticides are well known examples. Moreover, drugs used to treat infections of animals, or those added to animal feed to change the color or pigmentation of the skin, may be given for nontherapeutic purposes.

It is not unusual for a drug company to synthesize 30 to 40 new compounds each week, and one of the functions of pharmacology is to

111

test these compounds for various types of activity. They may, for example, be tested for their ability to cause sedation, to depress the central nervous system, or to increase the elimination of urine and body fluids—important in the treatment of heart and kidney diseases. Drugs are also screened for antiviral activity, for anticancer activity, for endocrine activity, for their ability to eliminate parasites from animals or people, and for anti-inflammatory activity (treatment of sprains, bruises, etc.).

Another function of pharmacology is to study the structure-activity relationship of various compounds. If the functional groups are changed or moved, the drug's actions may be changed. Also, saturation of unsaturated ring structures may change the drug's activity—an example is hydrocortisone, which has a greater activity than cortisone. Modifications of the basicity or acidity of certain compounds will determine antibacterial activity and will usually influence absorption from the gastrointestinal tract.

Since we live in an era in which drugs of all types are used considerably more than they were in previous periods, another function of pharmacology is to gather information about the interactions that drugs may have with other drugs. For example, if the antibiotic neomycin is administered to a person anesthetized with ether, there may be undesirable consequences. Neomycin has the ability to produce paralysis of the skeletal muscles and to interfere with normal breathing processes. Until this interaction was discovered some fatalities occurred in patients who received both ether anesthesia and neomycin. Another example of drug interaction is the absorption or inhalation of certain pesticides which alter the recovery time from anesthesia.

Branches of Pharmacology

There are several important subdivisions of pharmacology. Toxicology, the pharmacologic study of intoxicants or injurious substances, is concerned with the effects of poisons and their identification or detection. The toxicologist works to employ antidotes or drugs and procedures for treating intoxications. Toxicology laboratories assist in law enforcement and as centers for poison control. In the near future it appears that there will be environmental toxicology centers for monitoring and safeguarding our environment.

Another important subdivision is comparative pharmacology, concerned with drug responses in all species, ranging from single-celled organisms to man. An example of how differently a drug may act in different species is provided by a research project conducted to develop an anesthetic with a very short duration of action. It is desirable to have an anesthetic that will allow the patient to wake up and have full use of his faculties as soon as possible after an operation. A large amount of research was performed on dogs until it was thought that a good candidate compound had been developed to serve as a short-acting anesthetic. On the basis of excellent results in dogs, it was decided to test the drug in man. A male volunteer was anesthetized early in the morning. About 6:30 that evening his wife telephoned to find out when he would be home for dinner, and it wasn't until the next morning that the effects of the drug disappeared and the volunteer recovered from anesthesia.

Still another subdivision of pharmacology is clinical pharmacology, concerned specifically with the therapeutic use of drugs.

Historical Aspects of Pharmacology

The history of pharmacology is closely interwoven with that of chemistry. The first recorded mention of drug usage is dated at 2700 B.C., when a Chinese emperor classified and recorded all available drugs. In ancient Egypt drugs such as castor oil and opium were again listed and recorded. During the period of Greek dominance there was a change in the approach to disease from a philosophical attitude to a scientific basis. But it wasn't until the Renaissance (the 1500's) that chemistry really became involved. A Swiss physician, Theophrastus Bombastus von Hohenheim, called Paracelsus, wanted to use his knowledge of chemistry for something other than trying to synthesize precious metals. Paracelsus became the first person to use chemistry to discover drugs for the treatment of disease. One of his discoveries included the use of mercury for treating syphilis, an important social disease; but a limitation of this treatment was the undesirable toxic side effects. Shortly thereafter a French apothecary made a significant contribution by synthesizing an organic compound from potassium acetate and arsenous oxide. The organic arsenic compound had less inherent toxicity than inorganic arsenic and became a treatment for syphilis.

The first intravenous injection was an important development, and initiated a new and exciting approach to therapy. This took place about 1650 when the architect Christopher Wren and the physicist Robert Boyle inserted a quill in a dog's vein and administered a drug. Prior to this time all medications were administered by mouth or rectum, or were applied to the skin.

Another important milestone in pharmacology was reached in 1807 when Sertuner isolated a pure compound, morphine, from opium, a complex mixture.   That step took man more than 5,000 years to attain, and it wasn't until the early 1950's that the structure of morphine was identified and the compound synthesized.

The beginning of the modern age of chemotherapy occurred in 1910, when Paul Ehrlich developed a systematic approach to detect drug activity.   After testing 605 drugs, he discovered arsphenamine, which was promptly labeled "606."   Arsphenamine demonstrated antibacterial activity and had specific action against invading disease-producing bacteria.   Twenty-five years later, sulfanilamide, the first of the "wonder drugs" was discovered, followed by penicillin, streptomycin, and many other antibiotics.   Since then the various chemical sciences have played an increasingly important role in facilitating the synthesis of drugs that could be designed to be as effective and as safe as possible.

THE USE OF ANTIBIOTICS IN ANIMALS

Antibiotics and antibacterial drugs are used to treat diseases of man and animals.   In addition, many of these drugs are used for non-medical purposes in animal production.   Examples of drugs in non-medical and animal-production uses are penicillin, chlortetracycline, streptomycin, oxytetracycline, neomycin, sulfamethazine, and erythromycin.   There are also numerous combinations of these drugs used in animal feeds.

In 1971 approximately 500 million dollars was spent on drugs for animal production and animal diseases.   In the United States there are some 1,175 drugs and drug combinations allowed in animal feed.   Approximately 2.7 million pounds of antibiotics are used each year in animal feeds.   A large proportion of the drugs are used for nonmedical purposes.   They are added to animal feed with the aim of increasing the rate of weight gain, thus enabling the grower to market the animals sooner and with less feed.   Drugs are also administered at higher concentrations for therapeutic purposes in the feed, the drinking water, or by injection.   A large portion of the drugs used subtherapeutically are administered by nonprofessionals. Many of the drugs used in animal feeds are considered as treatments of choice for bacterial diseases in man.   When used in human medicine they require a prescription, but their use in animals is much less restrictive.   The drugs are readily available without prescription at feed stores, drug stores, hatcheries, hardware stores, etc.

Eighty per cent of the meat and eggs produced in the United States is derived from animals fed medicated feeds for nonmedical purposes. In 1968 approximately 87 million tons of feed was used to feed livestock and poultry. Of this total, 60 million tons was commercially prepared, and 40 of the 60 million tons contained drugs or medication; 30 of the 40 million tons, or 75 per cent of the medicated feed, required a withdrawal time.

The withdrawal time for animals fed medicated feed is an important aspect of animal production. A withdrawal time is the time that should elapse from the time an animal has last received a medicated feed or a drug until the animal is slaughtered for subsequent consumption by man. This varies from eight hours for penicillin to 30 days for dihydrostreptomycin. There are problems associated with withdrawal times. For example, in very large animal production units it is considered laborious and expensive to change the medicated feeding program to a nonmedicated feeding program for a rather short period of time. There is also the occasional problem that sick animals are sent to slaughter too soon--before the drugs are completely eliminated. The enforcement of compliance with drug withdrawal times is not readily accomplished with the current meat inspection methods.

Prevalence of Antibiotic Residues

Our laboratory has surveyed several classes of livestock and poultry for the presence of drug residues to determine if drug and feed additive withdrawal times were being followed. The prevalence of drug residues in animals at time of slaughter was determined for more than 5,000 animals in Illinois (which has better meat inspection procedures than some other states). The information obtained from urine samples was discouraging. Eight groups of swine were tested in Illinois during each of the seasons. Twenty-seven per cent of the 1381 slaughtered hogs showed positive results in tests for the presence of antibacterial substances. Ten per cent of the animals tested had penicillin residues. Beef cattle showed the lowest incidence of antibacterial residues of the domestic animals that were tested. In five groups of cattle tested, 9 per cent of the 580 animals showed positive results; two per cent of the cattle were found to have penicillin residues. Tests of urine samples from veal calves collected at slaughter consisted of six groups. Of the samples, 17 per cent had antibacterial residues; seven per cent of these were penicillinase-positive. Four groups of market lambs were tested: 21 per cent (68 or 328 animals tested) contained antibacterial substances, and four per cent of the animals were positive for penicillin residues.

The large numbers of animals with positive urine and fecal tests, the lack of visible injection sites, and the excretory and metabolic patterns of the commonly-used antibiotics indicated that most of the antibacterial residues were probably the result of oral drug administration. A strong possibility exists that drug withdrawal times are not being followed, but it could also be that the withdrawal times are inadequate or that the recommended dosage was exceeded.

Various tissues from domestic animals were also tested. The presence of antibiotics in the liver at the time of slaughter ranged from 16 per cent for lamb to 5 per cent for beef livers. The tetracycline group of antibiotics—chlortetracycline and oxytetracycline were most commonly found in liver and kidney tissue.

A question frequently raised concerns cooking. Does the process of heating meat destroy antibiotics? Some antibiotics are destroyed by heat—oxytetracycline for example. Other antibiotics, such as streptomycin, are not significantly altered during the process of cooking. Freezing has no effect in destroying antibiotic residues.

The degradation products and metabolites of the antibiotics must also be considered. For example, penicillin is degraded to penicilloic acid protein conjugates. These substances are a serious hazard because they have the ability to sensitize people to penicillin. It usually requires only a very small amount of the conjugate to develop sensitization within the body. The sensitizing substances may be ingested as food residues.

Public Health Concerns

The hazards associated with antibacterial drug usage can be considered from two standpoints. One point of concern is drug residues. The other point involves the ecologic changes the drugs produce on our external and internal environment when almost entire populations of domestic animals are exposed to these drugs.

If a drug residue is consumed, sensitization may occur or the bacteria in the gastrointestinal tract may become drug-resistant. Drug reactions range from minor skin rash to fatal anaphylactic shock. It is estimated there are 17 to 20 million people in the United States who are hypersensitive to antibiotics and other antibacterial drugs. Each year an estimated 600 fatal penicillin reactions occur in the United States.

In a Connecticut hospital study 1,000 patients were tested for drug hypersensitivity as they were admitted to the hospital. Fifteen per cent of the tested patients were found to be hypersensitive to some drugs. Penicillin reactions were the most prevalent, with 7.2 per cent of the patients being hypersensitive to that antibiotic.

Drug sensitization may be acquired by consuming the drug or its metabolite or degradation product. If you eat pork, the chances are approximately one in four that you have consumed an antibiotic, its metabolite, or a degradation product of an antibiotic or antibacterial drug. Such drugs could be classified as "occult drugs," those we consume without knowledge of their presence.

DRUG RESISTANCE

In England it has been reported that the development of drug resist- ance by bacteria in man's gastrointestinal tract is associated with the use of drugs in animals, resulting in a disease reservoir.

Bacteria which inhabit man's gastrointestinal or respiratory tracts may become tolerant or resistant to antibacterial drugs by various mechanisms. Some organisms become tolerant because of spontaneous mutational changes. A population of bacteria may become resistant because of the selective pressures of antibiotics administered as feed additives. The continuous presence of small concentrations of anti- biotics in feeds has an inhibitory or lethal effect on sensitive organ- isms, resulting in a larger population of remaining resistant organisms.

Another form of drug resistance may develop at a faster rate. Infectious or transferable drug resistance enables bacteria to become resistant to several drugs in a short period of time. Sensitive bacteria may acquire the resistance without being exposed to antibiotics. The resistance is acquired by contact with the extrachromosomal material from a drug-resistant bacteria.

The multiresistant organisms have probably acquired their resist- ance through the transferable drug-resistance process. The speed at which multiresistance occurs cannot be related to the other methods of resistance development via mutation and selection.

If one consumes meat or meat products containing antibiotics that are heat-stable and are not destroyed during cooking, bacteria in the gastrointestinal tract may become resistant to those drugs. One may also acquire resistant bacteria by direct contact with animals, live- stock or pets, that are hosts to resistant bacteria. Bacterial contami- nation of food may occur in the kitchen. For example, if raw chicken containing resistant bacteria of animal origin were allowed to remain on the kitchen counter, the bacteria could be picked up by contact with food such as bread, salads, or fruit which would not be subjected to high temperatures prior to ingestion.

The development of drug-resistant organisms is not restricted to the use of drugs in food animals. Indiscriminate drug use in man—for

example the use of penicillin to treat viral infections—may also contribute to the development of drug resistance. However, the use of
antibiotics and antibacterial drugs for nonmedical purposes in domestic
animals has made a substantial contribution to the prevalence of drug-
resistant organisms.

Drug resistance patterns and the prevalence of resistance transfer
factors (RTF's) which mediate transferable resistance in bacteria have
been studied recently in domestic animals and wildlife. The domestic
animals were subjected to routine production and health practices involving the presence of antibiotic pressures. Most of the antibiotics
were administered in the feed, less frequently in the water or by parenteral injection. The wildlife, on the other hand, had minimal exposure
to antibiotic pressures. They were trapped in the wild, but it is possible that occasionally a few of them might have consumed animal feed,
tissues, or feces containing antibiotic drugs.

A much higher percentage of bacterial isolates of E. coli were
observed to be resistant in domestic animals than in wildlife (Table I).
E. coli isolates from dairy cattle were 69 per cent resistant to dihydrostreptomycin, 56 per cent resistant to oxytetracyline, 27 per cent
resistant to ampicillin, and 12 per cent resistant to neomycin. The
E. coli isolates from wildlife contained a much lower prevalence of
resistant organisms. The high prevalence of resistant organisms could
be related to the prior exposure to antibiotic pressures occasioned by
the use of medicated feeds.

TABLE 1
Percentage of E. coli Resistant to Antibiotics

Antibiotic drug	Dairy cows	Dairy calves	Swine	Wild animals
Oxytetracycline	56	94	91	11
Dihydrostreptomycin	69	94	82	8
Ampicillin	27	25	37	3
Neomycin	12	12	3	8
Chloramphenicol	0	0	0	3

Multiresistant, RTF-bearing E. coli isolated from domestic animals
was generally more prevalent than sensitive, non-RTF-bearing E. coli
(Table 2). The prevalence of RTF-bearing E. coli was observed to be
much greater in domestic animals than in wild animals.

The prevalence of the RTF was from 17 to 92 times greater in
domestic animals exposed to antibiotics than in wild animals with

TABLE 2
**Prevalance of Resistance Transfer Factor
In Isolated** E. coli

| | *Per cent which transferred RTF* | |
Source of E. coli	E. coli	*Salmomonella typhimurium*
Dairy cows	52	50
Dairy calves	67	36
Swine	63	62
Wild animals	2	1

minimal or no exposure to antibiotics. Animals with minimal exposure to antibiotics had floras very sensitive to antibiotics and other antibacterial drugs.

The widespread use of antibiotics in domestic animals has resulted in almost complete populations of organisms becoming resistant to commonly used antibiotic drugs. The number of sensitive organisms has decreased, while resistant organisms have become predominant. No parallel situation, where populations of animals have been subjected to such antibiotic pressure exists.

Man can acquire some of the same diseases that infect animals. Some of these diseases are produced by organisms that are drug resistant. One might raise the question how the internist or the pediatrician would proceed if 95 per cent of his patients had been previously exposed to such drugs as penicillin, sulfanilamides, and tetracycline.

Remedies for the Situation

Some of the domestic animals slaughtered for human consumption contain antibacterial drug residues, with swine having the highest prevalence of residues and beef cattle the lowest. What can we do about it? We can begin by noting that there is a greater prevalence of antibiotics in our meat supply than in milk. This was not always so. At one time, 12 to 14 per cent of the milk was contaminated with antibiotics. In 1958, there was a concentrated effort by the milk industry and the federal and state regulatory agencies to do something about antibiotic residues in milk. Currently, antibiotic contamination is less than 0.5 per cent because of a cooperative inspection and law-enforcement program. The reduction in antibiotic contamination of milk was facilitated by the assessment of penalties and the enforcement of withdrawal times. A similar policy would improve the situation with regard to residues in meat. The improvement and broadening of meat inspection procedures and enforcement of regulations would help. Some states have assumed this task and have intensified inspection procedures of animals at the time of slaughter.

Drugs that are used for nonmedical purposes in animals could be restricted to those not also used for the treatment of disease. It would seem especially desirable not to use those drugs which are valuable for treating diseases of man.

In a recent issue of the *Medical Letter*, a publication sent to practicing physicians, 51 bacterial infections in man that required treatment with antibiotics were listed. The drug of first choice in 17 infections was penicillin. Penicillin was considered as an alternative drug in four of the remaining 34. Tetracyclines such as Aureomycin and Terramycin were considered as drugs of first choice in 10 of these diseases and as alternative drugs in 18 diseases. Streptomycin was considered a drug of first choice in five, and as an alternative drug in seven diseases. Erythromycin was considered a drug of first choice in four of the 51, and an alternative drug in 14 of the infections. All of these drugs are used extensively in animal feeds.

Drugs vary in their ability to induce resistance and share cross resistance. It would be desirable to use drugs as feed additives that do not have cross resistance with drugs that are used therapeutically or for treating diseases in man and animals and which would not contribute to the development of RTF or infectious drug resistance. Attention should also be directed to the synthesis of new drugs which can be used for nonmedical purposes as animal feed additives. It would be preferable that such drugs would not have antibacterial activity.

The problem can be greatly improved with discriminating use of the drugs currently available and by synthesis of new drugs with precise mechanisms of action and fewer side effects.

SUGGESTED READING

Huber, W. G.: The public health hazards associated with the non-medical and animal health usage of antimicrobial drugs, *Pure and Applied Chemistry,* 21:377, 1970.

Huber, W. G., *et al.*: Antibiotic sensitivity patterns and R factors in domestic and wild animals, *Arch. Environ. Health,* 22:561, 1971.

Huber, W. G.: The impact of antibiotic drugs and their residues, *Advances in Veterinary Sci. & Comparative Med.,* 15:101, 1971.

Huber, W. G.: Antibacterial drugs as environmental contaminants, *Environmental Science & Technol.,* 2:289, 1971.

THE DILEMMA OF DNA

Robert L. Sinsheimer

The dramatic event in Figure 1 is not a moon landing but a sperm landing. This is the critical moment for organisms relying on sexual reproduction—including man—the fertilization of an egg and the beginning of a new individual.

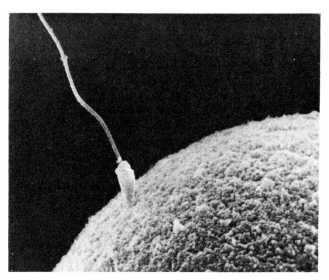

Figure 1: Contact of Arbacia sperm with egg. (Courtesy of Dr. D. Fawcett, Harvard Medical School.)

121

The essential role of the sperm is to carry in its head a cargo of DNA from the male parent to the egg, which holds a complementary cargo of DNA from the female parent. This process began in the dim reaches of geologic time, from which only tiny molecular traces remain and about which only myths may be known.

DISCOVERY

DNA was discovered in 1869 by Frederick Miescher. He was working in the laboratory of Hoppe-Seyler, the most famous German biochemist of that day. It is interesting that Miescher actually discovered *human* DNA, for he was studying the content of cell nuclei which he obtained from the leucocytes in human pus from a nearby hospital. After his initial discovery he turned to a more abundant source of DNA, which he found in salmon sperm.

Miescher's discovery of DNA—"nuclein", as it was then called—came only ten years after Darwin's publication of The Origin of Species, and only four years after Mendel's historic publication of the papers containing the basic laws of genetics. So within a ten-year period in the 1860's there occurred three of the most important events in the history of biology: the presentation of the theory of evolution, the revelation of genes, and the discovery of DNA. But as we know, another 75 years had to pass before the connection between these seemingly disparate discoveries could become evident.

The genes discovered by Mendel—the agents, the effectors of Darwin's evolution, although Darwin did not know it—had to have remarkable properties. How remarkable they were was not, and could not, be adequately appreciated until a good many years of research had passed. Not only did they somehow determine specific and complex traits—the color of a bean or an eye, the height of a plant, the shape of a fly's bristle, the texture of a mouse's skin (Figure 2); not only were they conserved unchanged from generation to generation to generation, (implying an extremely high precision of duplication); but occasionally a gene would change, to give rise to a modified, but obviously related gene—an allele—which could then produce a modification of the original trait, say a different eye color. This modified gene would in its turn be reproduced exactly, thereafter to continue to give rise to the modified trait. Evidently this process of stepwise gene change, with faithful gene reproduction between steps, has been going on throughout the whole course of evolution!

It taxed the imagination of those who pondered this scientific dilemma even to imagine a physical mechanism to account for these phenomena.

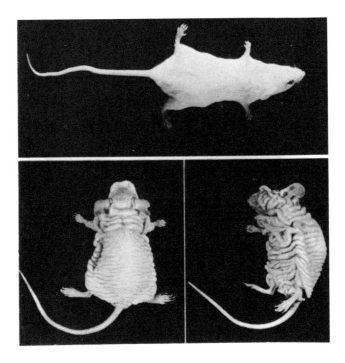

Figure 2: Comparison of normal and "rhino" mouse. (Normal mouse from Brachypodison: A Recessive Mutation of House-Mice, W. Landauer, Journal of Heredity, 43:293-298, 1952; Rhino mice from "Rhino," an allele of Hairlessness in the House-Mouse, Alma Howard, Journal of Heredity, 31:466-470, 1940.)

That DNA might be the solution to this dilemma was suggested very early, within 15 years after Miescher's discovery. In that period the chromosomes had been discovered, their duplication prior to cell division had been described, and thus their continuity from one cell generation to the next had been recognized. Furthermore, the essential role of the chromosomes in fertilization—the reformation of one nucleus after the union of the sperm and the egg cell—had been clarified. Already the chromosomes (Figure 3) had been assigned a role in inheritance.

It was also known, by staining techniques, that chromatin was a major component of the chromosomes, and further, that Miescher's nuclein was a principal component of chromatin. So in 1884 the zoologist Hertwig wrote "I believe that I have at least made it highly probable that nuclein is the substance that is responsible not only for fertilization but also for the transmission of hereditary characteristics." And in 1895 E. B. Wilson, the great American cytologist, wrote "Now chromatin is known to be closely similar to, if not identical with, a

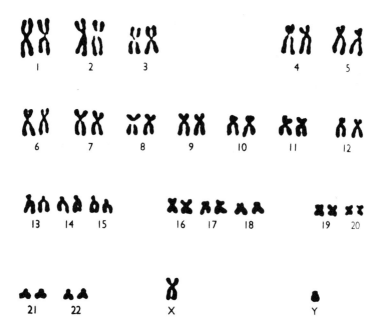

Figure 3: Normal human male karyotype. The chromosomes are grouped in pairs. While most pairs are unique, some can be distinguished only with very new techniques. These are often grouped together, as are 13-15, etc.

substance known as nuclein, and thus we reach the remarkable conclusion that inheritance may perhaps be effected by the physical transmission of a particular chemical compound from parent to offspring.''

But these were of course only correlations. There were genes and there were chromosomes and there was nuclein and they seemed to go together and so "perhaps" or "highly probably" there is a cause and effect. But scientific proof requires more than coincidence. And so the idea gained little credence. To suggest that DNA was the substance responsible for the remarkable phenomena of heredity merely solved one dilemma with another: how could DNA conceivably have the properties of a gene? Another 50 years of genetics was needed in order to prove directly that a gene was DNA; another 70 years of biochemistry was needed to show how DNA *could* be a gene.

Miescher himself did not fathom the idea of nuclein as the hereditary substance. In the early 1890's he was struck by the recently-discovered knowledge of stereoisomerism—that each carbon atom has four spatially distinct bonds and thus there are left- and right-handed stereoisomers. He conceived of a mode of inheritance based upon sequences of asymmetric carbons. He wrote, "With 40 asymmetric carbon atoms there can be a billion isomers[1]. . . . My stereochemical theory is better suited than any other to account for the unimaginable diversity required by our knowledge of heredity." His theory was ingenious; but nature chose other means.

It was 50 years later, in 1943, that Oswald Avery and two co-workers, Macklin McCarty and Colin MacLeod, first proved that a gene was DNA. This discovery is best described in a letter written in 1943 from Oswald Avery to his brother Roy. He talks about the problem he has been studying:

It is the problem of the transformation of pneumococcal types. You will recall that Griffith in London some 15 years ago described a technique whereby he could change one specific type through the intermediate R form. For example, type 2 pneumococcus went to type 3. This he could accomplish only in living mice. Dawson, with us, then reproduced the phenomenon in vitro. Later Alloway used a filtered extract. Once the reaction was induced the organisms continued to produce the type 3 capsule, that is, the change was hereditary. I have been trying to find out what is the nature of the substance in the bacterial extract which induces this specific change.

He goes on to talk about his chemical procedures, and then says:

When absolute alcohol is added dropwise to a concentration of about 9/10 volume there separates out a fibrous substance.... This substance is highly reactive in transformation and an elementary analysis conforms very closely to the theoretical values of pure deoxyribonucleic acid. Who could have guessed it?

Hertwig had been long forgotten, of course.

If we are right, and of course it is not yet proven, then it means that nucleic acids are not merely structurally important functionally active substances in determining the biochemical activities and specific characteristics of cells—and that by means of a known chemical substance it has been possible to induce predictable and hereditary changes in cells, which has long been the dream of geneticists.

Ten years later, in 1953, the famous double helix structure of DNA was deduced by Watson and Crick. This showed in one clear stroke how DNA could be a gene, how it could be sufficiently varied yet

---

[1] Actually, it would be a trillion.

specific, how it could reproduce, how it could mutate, and then re-produce the mutation—problems that had baffled geneticists for decades. The structure consists of two chains interwound helically. Each chain is composed of a linear sequence of subunits called nucleotides, of which there are four kinds in each chain. There is moreover and most importantly a complementary relationship between the two chains, so that whenever there is a particular nucleotide in one chain there is a complementary nucleotide in the other. This is illustrated in Figure 4.

In order to replicate the DNA molecule the two chains are in effect separated and each is used as a template upon which to build its com-plement, thereby producing two double helices, each identical to the old.

A mutation can be visualized as a change in the sequence of nucleotides along the DNA helix. The simplest form would be the replacement of one pair of nucleotides, say AT, by another pair, say GC; or simply by the inverse pair, TA. Another form of mutation would be simple deletion or insertion of a new nucleotide pair or, of course, of a tract of nucleotide pairs. Any such change once made would then be perpetuated by the same replication process already described.

FUNCTION

How can this DNA structure act to control the characteristics

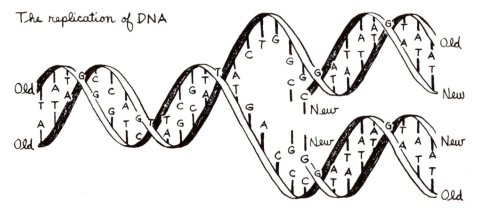

Figure 4: Replication of DNA.

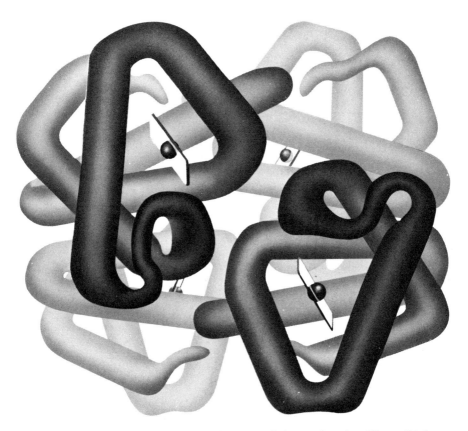

Figure 5: Schematic structure of the hemoglobin molecule. (From Dickerson, R. E., and Geis, I., The Structure and Action of Proteins, New York, Harper and Row, 1969.)

of a particular protein; for example, the hemoglobin in your red blood cells. Hemoglobin itself (Figure 5) is composed of an organic molecule: the heme group, an iron atom, and two types of protein subunits called alpha and beta chains. Each of these subunits is in turn a linear chain—folded in space—of monomeric units which are called amino acids. For example, Figure 6 illustrates the amino acid sequence of the β-hemoglobin chain. The gene for the beta chain of hemoglobin determines this specific sequence of 146 amino acids.

There is a simple code which relates the sequence of nucleotides in DNA to this sequence of amino acids in the protein; this is called the "genetic code." We now know what this code is and we know how the translation from DNA to protein is accomplished. Each sequence of three nucleotides in DNA is a *codon*, and specifies an amino acid. So a sequence of 438 nucleotides in DNA specifies the 146 amino acids of β-hemoglobin. In the cell the translation process is slightly

```
                         Val              10
        Val-His-Leu-Thr-Pro-Glu-Glu-Lys-Ser-Ala-Val-Thr-Ala-
                          20
        Leu-Try-Gly-Lys-Val-Asn-Val-Asp-Glu-Val-Gly-Gly-Glu-
                          30
        Ala-Leu-Gly-Arg-Leu-Leu-Val-Val-Tyr-Pro-Try-Thr-Gln-
        40                                       50
        Arg-Phe-Phe-Glu-Ser-Phe-Gly-Asp-Leu-Ser-Thr-Pro-Asp-
                                  60
        Ala-Val-Met-Gly-Asn-Pro-Lys-Val-Lys-Ala-His-Gly-Lys-
                          70
        Lys-Val-Leu-Gly-Ala-Phe-Ser-Asp-Gly-Leu-Ala-His-Leu-
             80                                  90
        Asp-Asn-Leu-Lys-Gly-Thr-Phe-Ala-Thr-Leu-Ser-Glu-Leu-
                                 100
        His-Cys-Asp-Lys-Leu-His-Val-Asp-Pro-Glu-Asn-Phe-Arg-
                         110
        Leu-Leu-Gly-Asn-Val-Leu-Val-Cys-Val-Leu-Ala-His-His-
             120                                 130
        Phe-Gly-Lys-Glu-Phe-Thr-Pro-Pro-Val-Gln-Ala-Ala-Tyr
                                 140
        Gln-Lys-Val-Val-Ala-Gly-Val-Ala-Asn-Ala-Leu-Ala-His-

        Lys-Tyr-His
```

Figure 6:   The amino-acid sequence of normal and sickle-cell hemoglobin. Normal hemoglobin contains a Glu at position 6, while sickle-cell hemoglobin has a Val at this position. (From Lehman, H. and Huntsman, R. G., Man's Haemoglobins, North Holland, 1966.)

more complex in its details. The nucleotide sequence in DNA is actually first transcribed into a nucleotide sequence in a similar kind of nucleic acid, called RNA. This is then translated by a complex machinery which reads the sequence of nucleotides and organizes the corresponding sequence of amino acids to make the protein (Figure 7). This process can now actually be seen also with the electron microscope (Figure 8).

Now the sequence illustrated is that of the normal beta chain of human hemoglobin. Some persons are carrying in their chromosomes a defect—an altered gene—for the structure of the beta chain of hemoglobin. This altered gene then produces an amino acid sequence which differs in one position (Figure 6) from that of normal hemoglobin. A glutamic acid has been converted to a valine. This is actually the consequence of a change of one base from an A to a T. This small genetic change results in a change in the properties of the hemoglobin so as to give rise to what is called sickle-cell hemoglobin. Instead of being the normal concave shape when deoxygenated, the red cell containing this altered hemoglobin looks like a sickle, is crecentic. This altered hemoglobin is much less soluble in the absence of oxygen

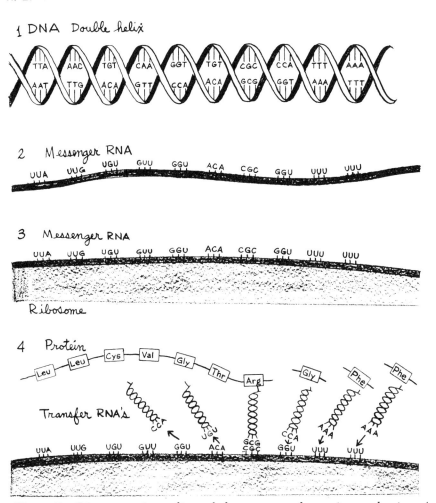

Figure 7: Diagrammatic outline of the process of protein synthesis. A messenger RNA molecule, transcribed from the helical DNA, is translated on a ribosomal surface, with the aid of transfer RNA molecules, to form a growing protein chain. (After Nirenberg, M. W., The Genetic Code: II, Scientific American, March, 1963, 80-94.)

and precipitates within the cell as a crystalline tactoid, changing its shape. The sickle cells are more fragile than normal cells, leading to anemia; they also occlude capillaries, leading to thrombosis. In an individual all of whose hemoglobin is of the sickle type, this is a serious metabolic problem—a genetic disease.

The newer knowledge of DNA has given us a deeper appreciation of the role of genes in the formation of all living organisms—including us—and thereby, as in the defective prescription for hemoglobin, an understanding of the serious consequences of a mistake in the genetic

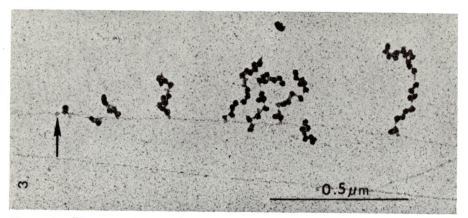

Figure 8: Electron micrograph of the process of protein synthesis. Strings of ribosomes are bound to the growing RNA chains, transcribed by RNA polymerase from the long DNA thread. (From Miller, O. L., Jr., Hamkalo, B. A., and Thomas, C. A., Visualization of Bacterial Genes in Action, Science 169:392-395, 1970.)

blueprint. An increasing number of human ailments have come to be recognized as the consequence of a genetic defect. It is estimated that approximately 6 to 7 per cent of all live human births carry an overt genetic defect. Six per cent is 250,000 births a year in the United States. The defect may become evident at various times throughout life (Figure 9). Since many of the defects take an early toll, the net

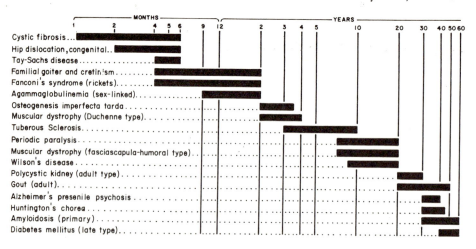

Figure 9: The age of expression of varied genetic defects. (From Aposhian, H. V., The Use of DNA for Gene Therapy—The Need, the Experimental Approach and Implications, Perspectives in Biological Medicine, 14:98-108, 1970.)

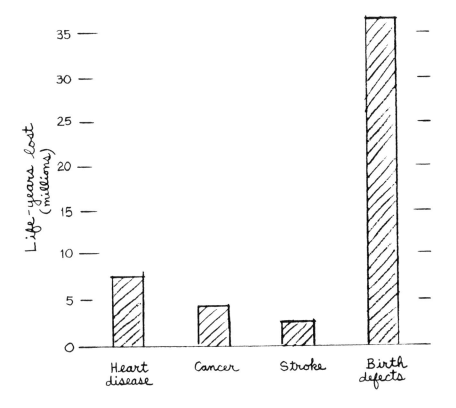

Figure 10: Comparison of life-years lost (per annum) from genetic and other diseases. (From Aposhian, H. V., The Use of DNA for Gene Therapy—The Need, the Experimental Approach and Implications, Perspectives in Biological Medicine, 14:98-108, 1970.)

effect of these genetic defects on the life-years lost to humanity exceeds that of many of the better-known diseases (Figure 10). It has been estimated that in this country approximately 36,000,000 future life years are lost each year as a consequence of birth defects, as compared to 8,000,000 from heart disease, 4,000,000 from cancer, or 3,000,000 from stroke. Another way to state the magnitude of the problem is, that genetic disease is estimated to cause 25 per cent of all hospitalization in the United States.

These genetic defects are of various kinds. Some—about one-half of one per cent of all births—are the consequence of an extra chromosome (Figure 11). Some, as in sickle cell anemia, are the consequence of mutations in a single gene. Others, as in diabetes and very likely schizophrenia, appear to be multigene defects, the consequence of a combination of mutations in two or more genes. Over 2,000 known

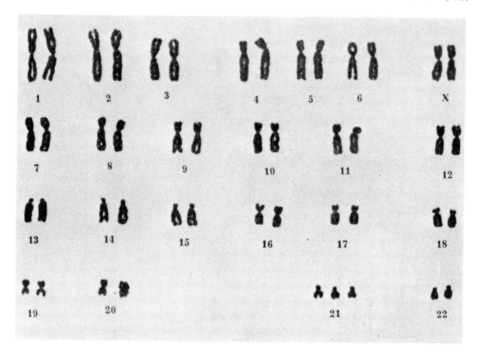

Figure 11: Karotype of Down's disease. Three chromosomes 21 are present, instead of the usual two. (From Ferguson-Smith, M. A. and Johnston, A. W., Annals of Internal Medicine, 53:359-371, 1960.)

human diseases are now recognized to be the consequence of inherited genetic defect.

As we come to appreciate the magnitude of this problem, and to understand, in scientific terms, its cause, it is natural for people to think of possible means to alleviate the problem; that is, in terms of repair of defective genes. Most defects are defects of omission—they reflect the absence of a needed component. Therefore, the easiest approach to gene repair would at this time seem not to be actual direct repair, which may be very difficult, but rather the addition of an effective gene (or the substitution of an effective gene) for the defective allele. Although we do not yet know how to do this, various schemes have been proposed which appear plausibly likely of success.

At this stage, however, we need a much deeper knowledge of the genetics of man. In many of the instances of genetic disease we do not yet know what gene is involved, or even on what chromosome the gene may be located. In fact, it is only within the last couple of years that it has been possible, by new staining techniques, to recognize definitively the various chromosomes of the human karyotype. With this new technique, and with the introduction of novel ancillary techniques, it is for the first time becoming possible to assign specific human genes to specific human chromosomes. Thus it has recently been determined that, for instance, the human gene for the enzyme thymidine kinase is located on chromosome #17. The mapping of the human karyotype is a most important task, and can only now begin to be approached. Many would consider it to be more important for the future of humanity than, let us say, the mapping of the moon.

In the discovery of DNA, and in the understanding of its central role in heredity, we have now achieved a conscious insight into the biochemical machinery underlying the entire process of evolution (Figure 12). After all these ages, a creature, man, has become aware of his origins and of how he came to be. And we are the first generation of man to have this knowledge.

POTENTIAL

But there is yet another chapter to this saga of DNA, and this chapter may become the most important of all. When we have learned to alter genes, we will have learned how to determine our own evolution. In that act we will have solved the scientific dilemma of DNA—but will have created the social dilemma of DNA. For what may we

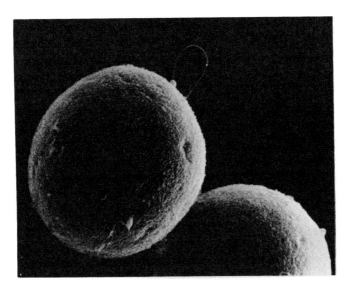

Figure 12: Contact of Arbacia sperm with egg. (Courtesy of Dr. D. Fawcett, Harvard Medical School.)

want man to be? Who knows what man may become as we choose our
way across the endless future? In today's troubled time, filled with
self-doubt, many deeply fear this prospect. As George Steiner has
written:

> It is as if the biochemical and biogenetic facts, potentialities
> we are beginning to elucidate, were waiting in ambush for
> man. It may prove to be that the dilemmas and possibilities
> of action they will pose are outside morality and beyond the
> ordinary grasp of the human intellect.

Do we really face an ambush? Or is this an epic opportunity? Is
this a dilemma too dense to penetrate, a potential too large to grasp?
Or is this the goal toward which evolution has been striving for five
billion years: to be in its product aware of its essence and thus to
rise above chance? To continue from this time on, the exploration of
the potential of life by means less harsh and in directions more varied?
To begin, slowly, with this imperfect instrument, *Homo sapiens*, the
application of forethought to evolution? And with forethought, con-
science?

These are most certainly profound questions. They merit both our
deepest thought and our highest motive. There are those who regard
all of this as a malignant human vanity and would have none of it; who
would deliberately halt all further research in this direction. My view
is that, in simple truth, here we are—at this juncture in our human
evolution—and we have really only two choices in this matter: to
proceed with all the wisdom we can develop, or to stagnate in fear and
in doubt. The choice seems to me to be: are we as a species to lead
a furtive, timorous existence in terror of our brute past, oppressed and
confined by our finite vision and our unfinished state? Or, using all
that evolution has given us, do we seek to find the way to a higher
state?

In *Homo sapiens*—self-aware, endlessly curious, endowed with the
capacity for logic, gifted with the opportunity for choice, and thus with
the burden of decision—something new has appeared on this small
globe. The next step for evolution is ours.

BLAME IT ALL ON MOTHER:

The Chemistry of Inherited Disease

Robert L. Switzer

Why should a chemist or a biochemist concern himself with genetic diseases? After all, the list of human miseries is enormous. In the disease category alone we have cancer, heart disease, and many forms of mental illness. We still have the misery of the common cold. On the other hand, inherited diseases are rare; the most common genetic disease in the United States is cystic fibrosis, which occurs with the frequency of about one in every 2,000 individuals. Phenylketonuria, a disease so common that most states require routine screening of new-born children for it, is found with the frequency of about one in every 10,000 newborn babies. In most cases inherited diseases occur with frequencies even less than this; frequencies of one in 100,000 or one in a million individuals are common. Some of these diseases occur with greater frequency in groups which have been somewhat isolated genetically. For instance, Tay-Sachs disease occurs in persons of Eastern European Jewish origin with the frequency of about one in one thousand. Sickle-cell anemia is really quite a common disease among black Americans. The question remains, though, why should a chemist be interested in such disorders?

Inherited diseases may affect few individuals, but the number of these diseases is large. At least 1,200 distinct inherited diseases are known, and there are certainly more to be found. There will also be found many examples of disorders in which inherited character-istics interact with certain environmental characteristics to produce

135

pathologies. So, collectively, the inherited diseases constitute a large group which affects very many people. Furthermore, the relative importance of these diseases has increased, and will continue to increase, as we vanquish the great infectious diseases which have affected mankind. To illustrate this, I have gathered some statistics. In 1900 in the United States, 150 out of every 1,000 newborn babies could not be expected to reach their first birthdays. Of that 150 per 1,000, 5 were fatalities resulting from inherited defects. Today we do much better. The infant mortality is now about 20 per 1,000 live births. However, 5 of those 20 deaths still result from inherited diseases, so that at present 25 per cent of infant mortality results from inherited defects. Relatively, the inherited diseases have become much more important.

Because inherited diseases are rare and numerous, it will be necessary to treat them a little differently than the great common killers, such as polio or diphtheria. If we are ever to deal with inherited diseases in a very effective way we will need a corps of specialists who have the facilities to diagnose them readily, know how to treat them, and are doing research in ways of preventing them. It is unlikely that the practicing physician will see very many of these diseases or will have the expertise needed to handle them properly. We need a national corps of specialists in genetic diseases to whom the practicing physician can refer. This is where the biochemist can contribute, because he can become a part of this research-diagnosis-treatment team.

In particular, the biochemist can contribute because the last quarter-century has seen an astonishing development in the understanding of the chemical basis of inheritance. We now have a rather good understanding of both the chemical mechanisms by which genetic information is passed from parent to offspring and the ways in which genetic information is expressed in the physical characteristics of the individual. I'd like to review briefly how this process occurs.

THE CHEMISTRY OF INHERITANCE[1]

A geneticist speaks of a *gene*, which is the fundamental unit of inheritance. A gene is that single genetic element which determines a single physical characteristic. We now know that what the geneticist calls a gene is made up of a very large molecule inside the cell called deoxyribonucleic acid, or DNA. We know that the information that a

---

[1] A more complete description of the process of gene expression can be found in Chapter "The Dilemma of DNA" by R. L. Sinsheimer, p. 121.

gene specifies is carried in the sequential arrangement of the various building blocks of DNA. DNA is a long, long chain made up of four different kinds of links, conveniently written A, T, G, C, for the four different types of nucleotides which are linked together in a nearly endless linear array. The sequence of these nucleotides can be highly varied. Such a long but continuously-varying sequence of nucleotides carries the genetic information. The way this is accomplished·is like the Morse code.

The Morse code uses dots and dashes and spaces, a three-letter alphabet, to specify more complex alphabets, the 26-letter alphabet of the English language. This is done by arranging the dots and dashes and spaces in different ways according to a previously agreed-upon dictionary. DNA does the same thing with its four-letter alphabet (A, T, G, C), but that information is transmitted by way of an intermediary molecule, called "messenger RNA." Messenger RNA uses a very similar four-letter alphabet (A, U, G, C) and is used to translate the genetic four-letter language into a 21-letter language, the amino acid sequence of a protein. The principle is exactly the same as used by the Morse code.

DNA not only allows genetic expressions through this kind of translation into amino acid sequences, it also allows faithful copies of itself to be made and passed from generation to generation. DNA is doubled at the time when the offspring forms, so that a faithful copy of the original sequence is transferred to the offspring. In higher animals there are two parents, both of whom contribute DNA to the offspring. The genetic information from each parent is combined at random, so that some of the DNA from the mother and some of the DNA from the father are combined to form the *phenotype* of the offspring. In most cases you can see, therefore, why children bear resemblance to both of their parents.

We have seen how chemical information can be passed from generation to generation. How does translation to the four-letter DNA language into the 21-letter amino acid language of protein permit the expression of genetic characteristics like the color of hair, or eyes, or the shape of a nose? The key lies in the protein. The genes specify what you and your offspring will become. But the protein specifies what you *are*. It is the proteins that completely specify what the characteristics of an individual will be. Proteins do this in two major ways. First, they are structural components of all cells and organs. For example, muscle cells are largely made of specific muscle proteins. The same is true of all other types of cells. Thus, the shape and character of a given cell is largely determined by the proteins making up that cell.

Far more important is the fact that most proteins are *enzymes*. To understand the role of enzymes one must realize that a living organism is not a static, finished object. It should rather be compared to an enormous house, which is constantly falling down and being put back together. The body of an adult individual changes very little in appearance, but it is not stationary at all in a chemical sense. A living organism is continually taking in food. This food is broken down through a long series of chemical reactions, releasing energy. This metabolic energy is necessary for various vital processes such as motion, conduction in the nervous system, and the resynthesis of new cells. Cells are constantly growing, dividing, dying, and being broken down and replaced. This dynamic process entails literally thousands of reactions. Each such biochemical reaction is a specific chemical reaction of the sort that one might study in organic chemistry. However, under the influence of enzymes, biochemical reactions differ in two ways from the kind of reaction that one can do at a lab bench. First, they are much more *specific*. Enzyme-catalyzed reactions proceed with a specificity that organic chemists usually cannot hope for. An enzyme will permit only one compound of many very similar ones to react. Second, enzymes catalyze reactions at rates that are undreamed of outside of biochemistry. Most of the reactions that occur in living cells would not proceed at all in the laboratory under temperature and pH conditions identical to those inside the body; yet these reactions proceed very rapidly in the presence of the appropriate enzymes. It is accurate to say that if an enzyme catalyzing a certain biochemical reaction inside the body is absent, that reaction will cease. This fact foreshadows what happens in inherited diseases.

What happens if something goes wrong? Suppose that during the translation from the four-letter alphabet of DNA to the 21-letter alphabet of protein the telegrapher falls asleep and misreads the message. Such accidents do occur in Nature—fortunately, very rarely. If a mistake occurs during the copying of DNA to form messenger RNA, or during the translation to RNA to protein, the change is usually not noticed by the organism. This is because there are many repeated rounds of translation, and the next round is likely to be correct. Thus, an occasional mistake is likely to be drowned out by the many subsequent accurate rounds of translation. If, however, a mistake occurs in the copying of DNA to form more DNA during the formation of offspring, a permanent mistake has been created. This permanent mistake is called a *mutation*. If the genetic information given to the offspring was copied incorrectly, all copies made from the defective DNA will also be made incorrectly. Both the offspring and any progeny of the offspring will express the alteration in their DNA in the protein made from that DNA.

Hence, the formation of a defective gene results in the formation of an altered protein.

Unfortunately, the altered protein is most likely to be a defective protein. Proteins have been so selected through eons of evolution that they are very nearly perfectly arranged for their function. Most of the random changes that could occur in that sequence of amino acids which specifies a functional enzyme are harmful ones. Thus, the most ordinary kind of defective gene that results from an error in DNA copying is a destructive error, which results in loss of enzymic function. There are exceptions, but in general a mutation results in the loss of some critical metabolic function.

CONSEQUENCES OF INHERITED ENZYME DEFICIENCY

Most inherited diseases are the consequence of a defective gene that results in the loss of the activity of some enzyme. What will be the consequences for the individual who has lost one of the many thousands of enzymes that he possesses? In general, they are disastrous. The most obvious consequence of loss of an enzyme will be

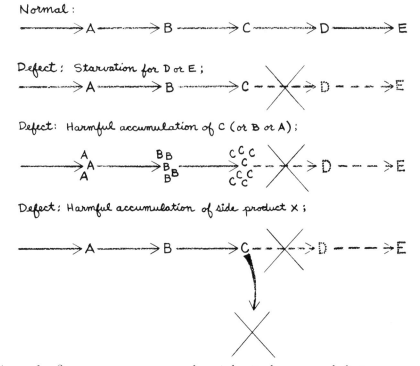

Figure 1: Some consequences of an inherited enzyme deficiency.

starvation for the product of the reaction catalyzed by the missing enzyme. An example is the inherited defect known as "albinism". An individual affected with albinism is missing the enzyme tyrosinase, which is necessary for the formation of the pigment of hair, skin, and eyes: melanin. These individuals have very white skin and white hair. It is not normally a serious matter for the affected person's health, although he is very sensitive to sunburn. This is a case of simple starvation for the product of a missing enzyme.

In other cases it is not the product of the enzyme which is a problem, but the missing protein itself. Such a case is the hemophilia with which the royal families of Europe were affected—the so-called "Curse of the Hapsburgs". Hemophilia is a disease in which one of about 12 important proteins of the blood is missing. These proteins act in concert when there is an injury to the individual, either external or internal, to bring about the formation of a clot. The clot prevents excessive bleeding. When one of these clotting proteins is missing because of an inherited defect, the blood of the affected individual cannot form clots readily. Even the smallest injury, a bruise or a cut, can become life-threatening, because the body is unable to prevent the continued flow of blood from the injury.

Another possible problem arising from the loss of an enzyme is the accumulation of the substance upon which the enzyme normally acts. An enzyme that normally passes this substance through a series of chemical reactions is missing, so that the substance accumulates. This accumulation may result in some sort of harm. An example of this is the group of diseases called the glycogen storage diseases. Glycogen is a quick energy source in the liver. Normally, glycogen is made from the supply of sugar in the diet, and can be used up very rapidly in response to stress. If the enzymes needed for the removal of glycogen are missing, glycogen is deposited continuously in the liver with a resulting gross malformation of the liver. The affected individual appears to have a very distended abdomen. Ultimately, the damaged liver begins to suffer in other vital functions.

Another common consequence of a missing enzyme is related to simple accumulation. The substance which is normally acted upon by the missing enzyme does not merely accumulate, but is also diverted into some secondary reaction. The flow of the accumulated substance through this second reaction may result in an accumulation of a toxic substance. This is the underlying mechanism of phenylketonuria (P.KU). In the case of PKU, affected individuals lack an enzyme needed to convert an essential amino acid, phenylalanine, into another essential amino acid, tyrosine. The lack of tyrosine might not constitute a problem, because tyrosine is available in the diet. However, the normal flow of phenylalanine into tyrosine is diverted to form the side product phenylpyruvic acid and a group of other phenylketone compounds, which accumulate in the nervous system and are thought to cause neurologic damage. Clearly, it doesn't take very much interference with the exquisitely balanced biochemical system of the cell to produce very severe effects.

PATTERNS OF INHERITANCE

It is worthwhile at this point to consider the patterns of inheritance found with this group of diseases. It is astonishing that two perfectly normal individuals with no history of health disorders can produce a child that is affected with some inherited defect. How can it be? How can you inherit something or pass on to your offspring something you yourself do not display? In fact, most of us probably carry within our genetic makeup the missing or defective genes that are necessary to specify one of the 1,200 or more inherited diseases that we have been considering.

The answer is that humans have not one gene for each characteristic, but two. If one has two genes, and one of them is inactive, not producing an essential enzyme, but the other gene is producing the enzyme, usually no harm results. We say that the inactive gene is *recessive,* and that the other, active, gene is *dominant.* Thus, the individual who has both a recessive (or defective) gene and a normal gene will be normal; his offspring will also be normal....

Except in those rare situations when he mates with another individual who has the same genetic makeup, that is, a healthy gene and a defective gene. In this case, one of three things can happen. Since genes are passed to the offspring at random from each parent, the offspring may have the same genetic makeup (one normal and one defective gene) as each parent; he can receive two normal genes, or he can receive two defective genes. If each parent has one normal and one defective gene, it can be predicted statistically that one out of four offspring will inherit the two defective genes. When there is no dominant normal gene to overcome the effect of the inactive recessive gene, the individual will lack some normal protein, usually an enzyme. This mode of inheritance, called *autosomal recessive,* is the one followed by many common inherited diseases. It should be clear that the genes for these diseases can be very widespread and yet not be expressed in most individuals. Only in those rare cases where two individuals who have the same recessive genetic effect marry and have children will we see the production of the disease. Even then, only about one-quarter of the children will be affected.

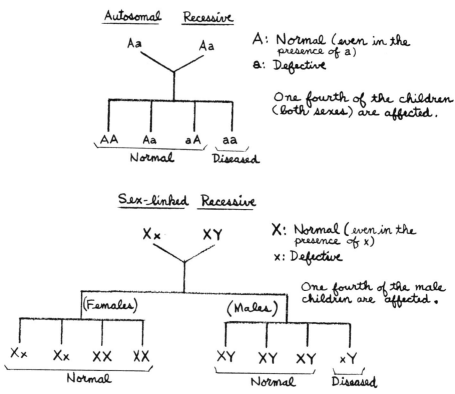

Figure 2: Patterns of inheritance in genetic diseases.

There is another fairly common pattern of inheritance of metabolic diseases. This is the type of inheritance which provoked the title "Blame It All on Mother". This type of inheritance is called *sex-linked recessive.*

Humans have two copies of every gene but this is not quite true of the genes that convey sexual identity. Here the situation is a little more complicated. Determination of sex is specified by many genes, but many of these genes are combined on the so-called X chromosome. Females have two X chromosomes, and hence two copies of the genes carried on this chromosome. Males possess a single X gene, but males have in addition a single "Y chromosome". The Y chromosome specifies the male characteristic, even in the presence of the X chromosome. The X chromosome carries more than the information necessary to specify female identity; it also carries many other genetic characteristics that are not related to sex determination.

If a defective gene happens to be located on the X chromosome, a different pattern of inheritance of the accompanying disease will be seen. Let's say a woman has one defective gene on the X chromosome.

Since these defective genes are rare, the other X chromosome will al-most always carry a normal gene, so that she will not have the disease that corresponds to the defective gene. However, when this woman has children, her sons will receive copies of her X chromosomes. Half of those that receive copies of their mother's X chromosomes will receive the one carrying the defective gene. Since the male has no second X chromosome, those sons receiving the defective chromosome will have the genetic disease. Thus, the pattern seen with this class of diseases is that the mother is almost never affected with the disease but one-half of her sons are. This is the case with some of the hemo-philias discussed earlier. Queen Victoria is probably the most famous of these female carriers of inherited diseases.

There are other types of inheritance, but they are less common. It should be clear that the recessive mode of action of these diseases favors their continuance throughout the population. Any dominant mode of inheritance would tend to cause the defective genes to be eliminated from the population if the consequences of that disease were very serious for the affected individual, because there would probably be no opportunity to marry and have children.

THE ROLE OF BIOCHEMISTRY

None of this has explained what a biochemist can contribute to medical problems arising from inherited disease. To answer this ques-tion, it will be useful to illustrate the major points with a specific inherited disease, with which we have done some work in our labora-tory.

The disease is called the Lesch-Nyhan Syndrome, after the two doctors who first described it. This particular syndrome is character-ized by mental retardation. The affected children also have a charac-teristic palsied movement which is known as chorioathetosis. Affected individuals tend to mutilate themselves—they have a compulsion to bite their hands and lips to the point of amputation. This is a very rare disease. Only about 150 cases have been diagnosed since the syn-drome was first described in 1964. The disease shows the pattern of sex-linked recessive inheritance that was described above. Only male children have been observed to have the disease. Its symptoms are so severe that the affected individuals normally do not live to adult ages. Finally, the disease has a characteristic that attracted the attention of biochemists—affected children have gout. To be more precise, they have hyperuricemia; they produce a great deal of a substance called uric acid. Uric acid is a waste product excreted in the urine by everyone, but in Lesch-Nyhan patients enormous quantities of it are produced. The urine of these children is not the clear yellow fluid that one might expect; their urine is actually cloudy with tiny crystals of uric acid. The kidneys are damaged by these tiny crystals. Most of the victims of this disease succumb to damage to the urinary system rather than other symptoms of the disease.

It was an attempt to treat the hyperuricemia of these children that led to the accidental discovery of the biochemical defect of this disease—a missing enzyme. Lesch-Nyhan patients were treated with a drug called azathioprine, which has been effective in reducing the accumulation and excretion of uric acid in gouty patients. It had no effect whatsoever on these children. The proposal was made that an enzyme that was probably required to convert azathioprine into an active form (an enzyme known as hypoxanthine guanine phosphoribosyltransferase) was absent in Lesch-Nyhan patients. This proved to be the case; although found in normal individuals, the enzyme was almost completely absent from Lesch-Nyhan patients. This has been found to be true in all cases of the syndrome which have been examined. Thus, when one has a way of measuring this enzyme, he can identify cases in which it is absent.

This is the first contribution of biochemistry to this type of disease—an unequivocal chemical tool for diagnosing the disease. Other individuals may mutilate themselves; other individuals are hyperuricemic; others have chorioathetosis or various other aspects of the Lesch-Nyhan Syndrome. However, if one has found a specific enzymic defect, he has a way of identifying the disease with real confidence. Since the biochemist is adept at devising specific and sensitive methods for measuring enzymes, he can help the physician to identify an inherited disease, and to avoid erroneous treatment which might be based on a faulty diagnosis.

The discovery of a biochemical defect in one disease may provide useful information in thinking about related diseases. The discovery of the enzyme defect of the Lesch-Nyhan Syndrome may help us to understand something about gout and some of the other diseases that are also characterized by excessive uric acid excretion. Indeed, the discovery that Lesch-Nyhan patients lack the enzyme hypoxanthine guanine phosphoribosyltransferase has led to the finding that some gouty patients have only 1/10 per cent as much of the enzyme as normal individuals. Such patients have none of the symptoms of the Lesch-Nyhan Syndrome, except hyperuricemia.

When the biochemical defect of an inherited disease has been identified, not only is a means of diagnosing the disease provided, but, in certain cases, we have also a means of detecting genetic carriers of the disease. In some cases it is possible to show that an individual carries the defective gene associated with a given disease, even if they have never had children. In the case of the Lesch-Nyhan Syndrome this is possible. You will recall that the defective gene for this disease is carried on the X chromosome. As a result, carrier mothers have cells in their bodies which carry the defective gene. In fact, not all the cells have the defective chromosome; for some as yet unknown reason, in each cell of the adult female one or the other of the two X chromosomes is inactivated. This means that some of the cells of the mother have the normal X chromosome and show the presence of this missing enzyme; other cells do not. We call this situation a *genetic mosaic*. Because of this it is possible to identify mothers who carry this lethal gene, but who are themselves not affected, by using specific biochemical tests for the missing enzyme.

This type of biochemical identification can also be used to find affected individuals who are not yet showing the symptoms of the disease. Children born with the Lesch-Nyhan Syndrome seem to be perfectly normal; they don't actually show the symptoms until after about a year of life. In many other inherited diseases the effects of a genetic defect may not be apparent for years. Gout, for example, rarely develops before the age of 40 or 50. In the case of Wilson's Disease, an ailment in which a copper-trapping protein of the blood is missing, the affected individuals usually don't show ill effects until five to ten years of age. The identification of such an individual by a biochemical test enables one to begin therapy before the patient's health has been damaged irreversibly by the genetic defect. This is of great medical value in the case of Wilson's Disease, in which copper from the diet accumulates and slowly poisons the liver. Affected individuals lack a protein called ceruloplasmin, which binds copper and prevents poisoning. If the absence of ceruloplasmin can be identified soon enough, one can administer a drug called penicillamine which will substitute for ceruloplasmin and carry the toxic copper out of the body, thereby preventing damage. But one has to know of the inherited defect before the individual has shown symptoms. A biochemical test for ceruloplasmin makes this possible.

Recently it has become possible to detect inherited disease in an unborn individual. Some adventurous obstetricians have learned how to determine the health of unborn infants by a procedure called *amniocentesis*. The technique is to introduce a long slender needle into the uterine cavity to puncture the placental membrane and withdraw some of the amniotic fluid that surrounds the fetus. The obstetricians were surprised to learn that, in addition to cells from the mother, there were cells in this fluid that were characteristic of the fetus. Apparently the fetus constantly sheds healthy cells. These fetal cells can be withdrawn, grown in culture, and studied. From these cells it is frequently possible to learn a great deal about the genetic characteristics of the unborn baby. For example, one can stain the chromosomes, search for the characteristic X and Y chromosomes, and determine accurately whether the fetus is a boy or girl. The procedure has certain risks, both to the mother and the unborn child, so it certainly is not justified simply to answer idle curiosity. However, when a family knows, or even suspects, that they carry the genes that specify a sex-linked disease, it is of great value to know the sex of an unborn child. In a sex-linked disease, it is known that half of the time the son will be affected, but the daughters never will.

But the technique is more powerful than that. If you know which enzyme is absent in a given disease, you can use the same analytical techniques that enable you to diagnose the disease in the affected individual, and test the fetal cells taken from the amniotic fluid. In this way one can determine whether or not the unborn child actually has the defect. This is possible with the Lesch-Nyhan Syndrome. Recently a paper in *Science* described two cases in which physicians detected the presence of the Lesch-Nyhan Syndrome, using amniocentesis to identify the disease in unborn fetuses at about 21 weeks of age. In the case of a disastrous genetic disease such as the Lesch-Nyhan Syndrome it is possible, and, I feel, morally allowable, to terminate a pregnancy at this stage.

The final point is perhaps most important of all. If we know the biochemistry of a disease, we should be able to design a rational treatment. How? Let us consider some approaches—some presently used, some purely speculative—to biochemical treatment or prevention of inherited diseases where the genetic defect, the absence of a specific enzyme, is known.

One approach would be to supply the missing product of an enzyme. We know the enzyme that is missing. We know the product that is missing. The individual is suffering because of starvation for the product. We can supply the missing product. This works in some cases. It works particularly well where the missing product is a small molecule or protein that circulates in the blood. In hemophilia, where a blood-clotting protein is missing from the blood, administration of a preparation of the missing blood protein directly into the bloodstream is often successful. But in most cases the missing product cannot be supplied so easily. You can't get it where it needs to be. Perhaps the product is required in the central nervous system. It is very difficult to get molecules, large or small, into the central nervous system where they may be needed to prevent damage.

Another approach to biochemical treatment of inherited disease is to prevent the accumulation of harmful substances resulting from the inherited defect. This might involve restricting the diet. In the case of phenylketonuria, affected individuals are poisoned by converting too much of their phenylalanine to phenylpyruvic acid instead of tyrosine in the normal pathway. As soon as phenylketonuria is identified, the affected individual is put on a diet which is very restricted in phenylalanine, so that the excessive accumulation of a product from phenylalanine metabolism can be avoided. Drugs can be used for the same purpose. A common method of treating gout (excessive amounts of uric acid) is to give a drug called allopurinol, which inhibits some of the reactions that form uric acid.

In principle, one should be able to cure an inherited disease by supplying the missing enzyme itself. I don't know of any situation where this has proven to be successful in sustained therapy. The problems are complex. The body does not like foreign proteins; it destroys them. If the missing enzyme were put into a pill and swallowed, the acids and the enzymes in the stomach would very quickly destroy the enzyme. Thus, this route is not available except in unusual situations. If one places the missing enzyme directly into the bloodstream, the body usually identifies the protein as a foreign protein and it forms antibodies to it. This destroys the enzyme and may make the patient extremely sensitive to the foreign protein, so that he must stop taking it. In any event, the enzymes generally have to go beyond the bloodstream; they must go into the cells, the places where they actually function. The enzyme may be required only during a period of development when the individual is not yet born or during an early period of life. Or the enzyme may be required only in certain cells or tissues and be harmful in other cells. The fact is that we aren't very sophisticated at getting enzymes into cells.

Another approach to inherited disease introduces a field that has received a certain amount of controversial attention. This area has been called "genetic engineering" or "genetic intervention". The problem of inherited disease is usually a defective or missing gene. Could one place the proper *genes* into the cells and allow the normal body machinery to translate that gene into the protein? This approach would have the cell solve the problem of getting the enzyme where it belongs—a problem that cells obviously know how to solve. The problem would then be how to get the gene into the cells, and when to do it.

One approach has been called somatic alternation. In this case one would attempt to introduce healthy genes into the individual after one learns that he is affected. The clearest idea of how to do this, it seems to me, comes from researchers who have been studying the effect of bacterial viruses on bacterial cells. In bacterial genetics one can put a gene, almost any gene desired, into a bacterial virus. The virus can then invade a bacterium, into which it vanishes. Inside the cell the virus goes into a quiet state, where it does not cause harm to the bacterial cell and yet where the genes that were brought in with it are expressed by the bacterial cell. One can bring about a genetic transformation of bacterial cells in this way.

In principle, one should be able to do the same thing with animal viruses. One should be able to build desired genes into animal cells. It has not yet been possible to do this. The animal viruses are much more complicated creatures than the bacterial viruses. We know a great deal less about how they invade cells and what happens to them when they go inside the cells. Animal viruses do seem, in some cases, to undergo the same kind of disappearance, but it is unknown whether or not they can carry foreign genes in this way. Of all the means of genetic intervention this seems to me to be one of the most promising, but it may be a long time before it is actually possible to use it in treating disease.

Another approach would be to alter the germ cells, the first two cells of the human creature at the moment of conception. One might somehow alter the genetic characteristics of the DNA of the sperm cell or the ovum, allow these to combine, and to develop into healthy individuals. This is a staggering task in terms of what we now know. The models that we can derive from bacterial genetics don't help us very much. There is substantial question in my mind as to whether this approach will ever be medically significant.

I would like to close on a sober note. The kinds of genetic manipulation of human cells we have been speaking of are intended to aid in the alleviation of the suffering caused by inherited disease. The ability of biochemistry to contribute to this in only beginning. Unfortunately, as the social usefulness of a new scientific field increases, so also does the potential for use of the same scientific knowledge to increase human suffering. It is perhaps unlikely, but certainly conceivable, that the same techniques of genetic intervention that might be used to control inherited diseases could be used to invent gruesome weapons for biological warfare. This warning is not intended as a call to stop research on genetic intervention in higher animals. That would be neither possible nor desirable. Rather, it is a call for vigilance and the highest humanitarian standards of conduct from both the scientific community and informed laymen. The biochemist has long claimed that the research he does for "the fun of it" is of great value to mankind. As this proves to be true, he will acquire a new and very great responsibility—to do all he can to see that his work is used for human welfare rather than human suffering.

SUGGESTED READING

Danes, B. S., Genetic Counseling, *Medical World News*, Nov. 6, 1970,
     p. 35.
Davis, B. D., Prospects for Genetic Intervention in Man, *Science* 1970,
     1279, 1970.
Stanbury, J. B., Wyngaarden, J. B., and Fredrickson, D. S., The Meta-
     bolic Basis of Inherited Disease, 3rd. ed., New York, McGraw-
     Hill, 1972.

BUTTERFLIES OF THE SOUL

Drugs and Mental Illness

William O. McClure

As most of you are aware, we arbitrarily divide mental illness into two categories: neuroses and psychoses. Neurotics are the usual people one sees in the street—those who get along pretty well within their culture. In contrast, psychotics are a little bit further out than the rest of us. They cannot cope adequately with the stresses of modern civilization, or at least with their culture. The psychotic is the person to whom we must address ourselves.

A large number—probably over 100—of different types of psychosis have been defined. Fortunately, within the last ten or fifteen years this number has been reduced to a degree which is quite encouraging to those who hope to treat these diseases. We now class about 80 per cent of all psychotics as schizophrenics. The remaining 20 per cent fall in a number of less well-defined classes.

How many people does the figure of 80 per cent actually indicate? About half of the total hospital beds in the United States are filled with the mentally ill. This accounts for about 17 million people. An additional 40 million people regularly take physician-prescribed tranquilizers for some level of mental illness. A large number of those, were it not for the tranquilizers, would probably require hospitalization or some other form of in-house treatment. Clearly, we deal with a large number of people.

This is also an immense problem from a financial standpoint. The amount of money that the United States pays every year in order to treat its mentally ill people is in excess of 3 billion dollars, without including the amount lost through work-time absence. Since these figures neglect several considerations, such as the number of people not under a physician's care, the actual number may be considerably larger.

Depressing though these figures are, the actual problem will almost certainly become worse. The number of those who have succumbed to schizophrenia has increased briskly during the past half century. The nature of the increase is interesting, as it probably has a great deal to do with increased population pressure. As population density rises, two complicating factors affect the observed incidence of schizophrenia. First, with more people living close together, the more people there are observing any one, and the more obvious any aberrant behavior becomes. A farmer in southern Illinois can probably function effectively even with rather severe schizophrenia as long as he can plant and harvest his crop, even if he has to hop on what he thinks is a dragon to do it. If he can get his crops to market, he is successful. An equally disturbed person living in New York City is less likely to be successful, because his hallucinations are much more real to people around him. Second, the more complex a society becomes, and the more crowded it becomes, the less it can accommodate deviant behavior. Under these conditions, it is even more important that people whose behavior is not "normal" be somehow modified so as not to strain too strongly the delicate fabric of society. These two factors taken together may account for much of the apparent rise in mental illness.

The most obvious question is: how can we treat these people? In many ways, the treatment of mental illness has changed remarkably little during historical time. The Egyptians, who had apparently not made the connection between behavior and the brain, treated the brain rather lightly. Upon death, Egyptians were subjected to having their skulls opened and the brains scattered on the ground. The vile-smelling, brownish-gray substance found in the cavities of the skull was considered part of the garbage disposal system of the body—hardly a fitting accoutrement for people travelling to the after-world. Being unaware of a rather vital flaw in their logic, the Egyptians were unable to treat their mentally ill effectively, praying only that the gods who possessed these people would leave them.

Numerous other cultures, some much earlier than the Egyptians, were more sophisticated in this regard. They were aware that the brain was strongly connected with behavior, probably because they observed what happened to people after serious head injuries. People of these cultures formulated the relationship between mental illness and the brain in a number of different ways. Some thought the brain accumulated excess heat: others believed the brain collected an excess amount of pressure from one source or another. Many cultures believed the brain collected an excessive number of spirits. These people attempted to relieve the undue pressure by opening the skull and allowing the causative agent to issue forth. The openings were usually accomplished without anasthesia. Remarkably enough, they were not always fatal. The well-healed skulls of people in which such a wound has been made are found in archeological remnants from many very early cultures. Because opening the skull would help to relieve the internal pressure of brain tumors, with which some of these patients were probably afflicted, a certain degree of relief may have accompanied the surgery.

In the early 1900's hypotheses about the cause of mental illness began to reflect more modern thinking. There is a lovely quotation from the great Spanish anatomist, Ramón y Cahal, who actually spent a portion of his scientific life looking "in the flower garden of the gray matter for the butterflies of the soul"; thinking there to find nerve cells with strange and delicate shapes with which might be associated the cause of mental illness. We now know that such cells do exist in vast numbers, but we do not yet know whether they have anything to do with mental illness. Rather, our modern butterflies have chemical forms, as will be discussed later.

At about this same time, psychoanalysis was introduced as a means of treating the mentally ill. Psychoanalysis works very well for some of the mentally ill; unfortunately, it doesn't work for all, or even for most, of these patients. Furthermore, another problem was apparent, even in the early part of this century: the mentally ill were increasing in number, and were increasing relatively rapidly. Freud was aware that analytic help could not be supplied to more than a limited number of patients, partly because the process usually requires long hours of contact, and partly because the training of analysts is itself a lengthy process. He felt that an ultimate cure for mental illness must come from the laboratory of the chemist, and stated that behind every successful psychoanalysis stood a man with a syringe who, hopefully, would be able to take over the psychoanalytic duty. Unfortunately, the man with the syringe was not to appear for some time.

Through the 1920's and 1930's in the United States, we continued to treat the huge number of psychotics by a method that has apparently been relied upon since time immemorial: we put them in small boxes and closed the lids, operating on the assumption that to protect society from the offense of their aberrations, and to protect the ill from themselves, institutionalization was the only feasible remedy. The familiar phrase, "Out of sight, out of mind," may never apply as well as it does to our treatment of the mentally ill in this part of our history. We are now, perhaps, beginning to repay our debt to those whom we incarcerated. During the last two decades we have begun to treat the mentally ill more effectively. Much of the improved treatment is due to advances in our knowledge of the effects of drugs upon mental illness.

RAUWOLFIA

The origins of chemotherapy for schizophrenia are to be found as early as 2500 B.C. in a Hindustani document called the Rig Veda, which described a number of medicinal plants. Later Indian documents amplified on the uses of those plants. One, the Charka Samhita, written about 1600 B.C., was a remarkable handbook for the practicing physician. In this document are listed over two thousand remedies for different medical problems. Almost all of these remedies rely on drugs of plant origin. The plants necessary are described in detail great enough that one can still, after going back and reading the original text, recognize many plants. One of these is snakeroot: a gnarled, twisted shrub found in almost all tropical countries, widely used by natives to treat a variety of diseases. Snakeroot was reputed excellent for treatment of snake bites, for the treatment of poisoning of several different types, and, most important to us, for treatment of maniacal forms of mental illness, which primitive people saw occasionally.

After use for thousands of years, snakeroot almost became lost from the Indian literature in the early 1920's. India's native practitioners began to be replaced by modern medical people, most of whom ignored vegetable remedies taken from the old times. Money was not available with which to confirm the utility of the many remedies of the Charka Samhita. Fortunately, the Medical Research Council of India came to the aid of a number of physicians with the first of the Indian grants-in-aid to scientific research. Supported by these grants, research was carried out on many of the remedies in the Charka Samhita, including snakeroot. As a result, by the middle 1940's over a million Indians were being treated with snakeroot every year for a variety of complaints ranging from headaches to mental illness.

It is ironic that it was as a remedy for headache that snakeroot was introduced into the Western world. As early as 1563 a Spanish physician, Garcia de Orta, first wrote about the efficacy of snakeroot for treating headaches, as well as other maladies. His claims for the drug were so extreme that no one believed them possible. For that reason, the use of the plant was banned from the West—by neglect rather than decree—until 1949. In that year an Indian physician carried out careful studies at a hospital in Bombay. R. J. Wakil found that

headaches caused by high blood pressure could be dramatically re-
lieved by the use of snakeroot (now known as rauwolfia, the name
given by Linnaeus). Published in a British heart journal, the work
attracted the attention of Robert Wilkins, director of the Hypertension
Clinic of the Massachusetts Memorial Hospital, who introduced rauwolfia
into modern American medical practice. In 1952 Wilkins published his
major finding on rauwolfia: the compound was a mild hypotensive
agent—an agent which slightly reduces blood pressure, and which in
this way functions effectively to reduce the severity of some types of
migraine headaches.

Wilkin's paper started a landslide. Rauwolfia, administered for
the treatment of hypertension, acted to make patients very sedate.
They were relaxed, content—even executives who suffered from high
blood pressure became relaxed, often to the point of not functioning
normally, despite relief from their headaches. The tranquilizing effect
was noticed very quickly by psychiatrists. So quickly, in fact, that by
1953 the use in the United States of electroshock therapy for treating
psychotic patients had in 90 per cent of cases been replaced by treatment with rauwolfia, or with compounds purified from the plant. By
1957 at least 1700 papers on the effects of these chemicals, isolated
from rauwolfia, had appeared. The snakeroot plant taken from India
had revolutionized the treatment of mental illness. In a conference
held in 1962 by the New York Academy of Medicine the closing address,
given by the president of the Academy, stated that rauwolfia had for
the first time in history removed the taint of horror from mental treatment and mental institutions. For the first time it was possible to
consider the treatment of mental illness on a rational basis, with the
thought that mental patients could eventually be brought back into
normal society.

Because of the spectacular success of rauwolfia, a tremendous
amount of work and money were poured into improved drugs. Tauwolfia
is a crude plant product, made up of a mixture of many complex compounds. Presumably only one, or a few, of these compounds are responsible for rauwolfia's therapeutic effects. To prepare more potent
medicines, and to study the action of the drug in the laboratory, it was
necessary to isolate the active substance from the powdered root. The
first compounds isolated, by Indian chemists, showed no activity
against mental illness. In 1952 Emil Schlittler, of the Ciba Laboratories in Switzerland, succeeded in isolating from rauwolfia an alka-
loid which he named reserpine (Alkaloids are nitrogen-containing compounds of plant origin, Figure 1). Reserpine has nearly all the tranquilizing properties of rauwolfia. The complexity of reserpine is clearly
an organic chemist's nightmare. It has, nonetheless, been synthesized.

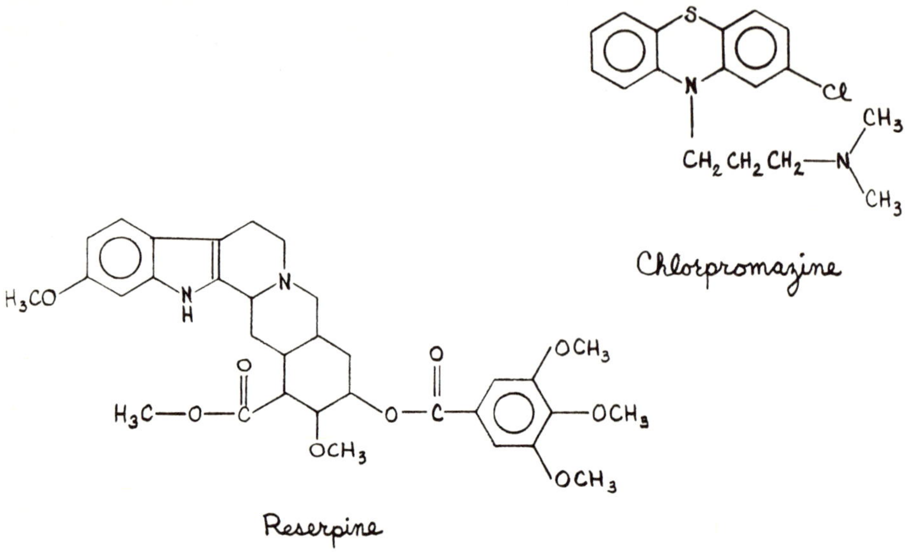

Figure 1: Structures of reserpine and chlorpromazine.

The feat was accomplished in 1956 by R. B. Woodward, of Harvard University, and has resulted in the commercial availability of synthetic reserpine. The synthesis of a compound of this size and complexity is accomplished neither easily nor cheaply. At the present time it is not clear whether synthetic reserpine will be less expensive in the long run than reserpine isolated from rauwolfia. But, whichever wins out, the price of reserpine has already fallen to the point that it now is used very widely for treating mentally ill patients.

CHLORPROMAZINE

The identification of reserpine led to a search for similarly effective compounds which had been synthesized directly in the laboratory. Prior to the early 1950's a number of compounds had been synthesized here which, like reserpine, belong to the pharmacological class of tranquilizers. None was as effective as reserpine. In 1952 a compound originally marked as an antihistaminic drug began to achieve fame as a tranquilizing agent. This compound, chlorpromazine, has the structure given in Figure 1. Chlorpromazine is one of a number of compounds which possess approximately equal efficacy in treating mental disease. Since the introduction of these first compounds, several related ones have proven effective and are now used.

Before the advent of rauwolfia and chlorpromazine, theories concerning the causes of mental illness were nearly without number. That the symptoms of the illness might be alleviated by administering a drug suggested that, in schizophrenia at least, the illness was related to a biochemical deficiency. It became possible to consider schizophrenia as a disease of the brain rather than a disease of the mind. This concept was important, for it meant that mental illness might be treated as any other disease. Although mysterious errors in the functioning of the mind might be difficult if not impossible to identify, an error in the chemical balance of the brain might be localized more easily. Research in biochemistry was beginning to uncover the fabled butterflies of Ramón y Cahal.

Genetic lines of scientific evidence also suggest that chemical factors are involved in schizophrenia. It seems fairly clear from case histories that the probability of a twin's having schizophrenia is high if his identical twin has the disease. There are available a number of other lines of evidence—some more convincing, some less—which also lead to the conclusion that schizophrenia is a malady to which a genetic pre-disposition is inherited. Given the proper environmental stress, a person with this pre-disposition can develop the full-blown disease.

The environmental element of mental illness is in part related to increasing population density. Despite the problems associated with crowding, we are becoming a more urban population all the time. Mental illness will increase as long as our cities continue to grow in size. We must find more effective ways of dealing with this problem than the drugs we now possess. As effective as the tranquilizers are in alleviating mental illness, they have definite shortcomings. In some patients side effects limit use; in other patients little relief is seen; and so on. It seems clear that more and better therapeutic agents will be necessary to complete our conquest of mental disease.

CAUSES

One facet of the search for better therapies is investigation of the causative factors of schizophrenia. The first modern hypothesis of the causative factors of mental illness was E. Kraepelin's suggestion in 1892 that mental illness is associated with a phenomenon he termed auto-intoxication. We continue to call this fascinating idea the autointoxication hypothesis. The hypothesis, which explained very well the evidence then available concerning mental illness, continues to fit equally well the evidence we have collected today. The autointoxication hypothesis states that a schizophrenic suffers an error in metabolism such that he creates, in his own body, a chemical compound which produces hallucinations, or which gives the appearance of physical or mental illness. Kraepelin based his observation on a report of research by Bouchard, of Paris. In 1887 Bouchard had carried out experiments in which he injected urine from schizophrenic patients into rabbits. He found that urine from schizophrenics killed rabbits, while urine from normal patients did not. These results suggested that in the urine of schizophrenics there was some chemical compound which was absent in normal urine. These experiments provided a basis five years later for the autointoxication hypothesis.

Since that time a number of chemicals have been suggested as the compound mediating the autointoxicated response in schizophrenia. There is an element of humor in these studies. For example, allow me to paraphrase pages taken from a book now commercially available. It has been stated that serum from schizophrenic subjects is more lethal to mice than serum from normal subjects (six references are given); is more toxic to certain cells in tissue culture (three references); produces an effect in rabbits which causes the glucose level in the blood to increase (three references); inhibits the growth of plants; leads to aberrant rope climbing in untrained rats; when injected into spiders causes the spinning of strange-shaped webs; may contain a factor which destroys red blood cells; etc. Bile from schizophrenic subjects, but not bile from normal subjects, has been reported to produce differentially catatonic symptoms in mice, pigeons, and cats; and so on. Unfortunately, for every paper in which these effects are reported, an equally careful study has been carried out which concludes that they do not occur. On the following pages of the same book, another set of references gives the negative side of the same argument.

These studies, ingenious though they are, have not demonstrated the presence in schizophrenics of any chemical which would verify the autointoxication hypothesis. The fundamental idea of the autointoxication hypothesis, however, is still very much with us. Justifiably so, for the inherent simplicity of the hypothesis renders it still very attractive. We can prove the hypothesis correct when we find the right compound, but can prove it incorrect only by ruling out each of the chemicals suggested as candidates. With the incredibly large number of chemical compounds which are found in the brain of a human being, it seems nearly impossible ever to prove the autointoxication hypothesis wrong, except by postulating an alternative hypothesis that *can* be proven.

Despite its shortcomings, therefore, the autointoxication hypothesis continues to shape much of the research concerned with mental illness. Many compounds have been suggested as chemical mediators of the hypothesis.   H. Osmond, in 1954 reported an interesting example of serendipity when he treated asthmatic patients with oral doses of the hormone epinephrine (adrenalin).   Unfortunately, the epinephrine which he used had been sitting on the shelf for some time and was discolored—it was tinted slightly brown in color.   The patient recovered from the asthma, but while doing so exhibited behavior that Osmond recognized as characteristic of mild schizophrenia.   Having some of the colored epinephrine left, he was able to analyze it chemically.   The most interesting compound found is called adrenochrome (Figure 2). Adrenochrome can be produced, in a series of reactions, from epinephrine, a compound which normally occurs in tissues.   Adrenochrome is a hallucinogen—that is, when adrenochrome is injected into most people, they suffer hallucinations, and exhibit behavior similar in some respects to that seen in schizophrenics.   Adrenochrome can in turn be converted to a second compound, adrenolutin.   Both adrenochrome and adrenolutin are found in discolored epinephrine, and both produce hallucinations.   It is not clear whether one, or the other, or both, are present in schizophrenics—at least, it wasn't clear when Osmond published his results.   In the last few years a number of studies have been carried out with urine, with serum, and with other tissue fluids from schizophrenics.   The present evidence suggests that neither adrenochrome nor adrenolutin is responsible for autointoxication.   However, the lines of evidence in this case are not as clear-cut as one would like.   These compounds, I think, remain possible chemical candidates for the autointoxication hypothesis.

   In the continuing attempt to identify the active component of schizophrenic urine, another class of possible autointoxicants was isolated.   After chromatographic separation[1], urine from schizophrenics

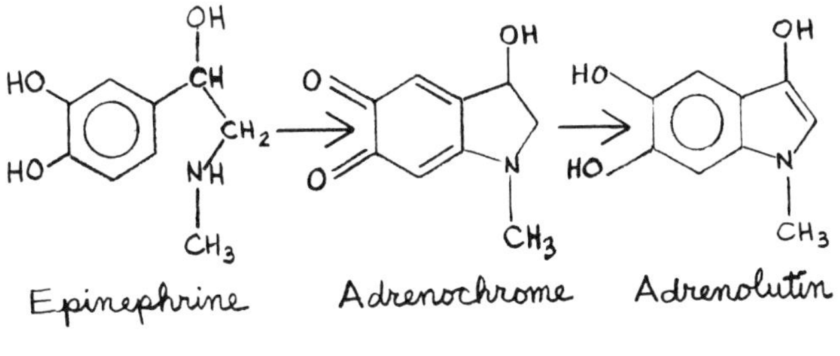

Figure 2:   Formation of adrenochrome and adrenolutin from epinephrine.

---

[1]Chromatography is a simple, rapid, yet very effective technique for separating the components in a mixture of chemicals. After chromatography on paper, separated material can be visualized as discrete colored spots by treating with proper reagents.

produced a pink spot not observed in normal urine. The pink spot was immediately pronounced by many researchers as the cause of schizophrenia. Pink spot isolated from the urine of a number of schizophrenics and injected into rats and other experimental animals did actually induce in these animals a state resembling schizophrenia. The structure of the pink spot substance, determined several years ago, is given at the left of Figure 3. Publication of the structure excited tremendous interest because of its similarity to the structure of mescaline, the hallucinogen isolated from the peyote cactus. The chemical similarities between the pink spot substance, dimethoxyphenethylamine (DMPEA), and mescaline, led very quickly to the suggestion that DMPEA might be the agent causing autointoxication. It probably is not. There have now been a number of studies done on pink spot with conflicting results. There exist two flaws in the case of DMPEA as the active material causing schizophrenia. First, DMPEA is found in normal subjects as well as in schizophrenics. The reported absence of DMPEA in normal subjects was due to inadequate analytical techniques. Second, careful chemical analysis of the pink spot showed that not only DMPEA but several other chemicals were found in this area of the chromatogram. Ironically enough, other major constituents of the pink spot are products of the metabolic breakdown of chlorpromazine used to treat schizophrenics. This only serves to emphasize the degree of precision required in studying the chemistry of biological systems. Furthermore, all chemical techniques are proportionately more difficult to carry out in complex biological samples. Much important chemistry, particularly analytical chemistry, must be done before biological materials can be properly studied.

BUFOTENINE

A third possible endogenous hallucinogen is bufotenine. This compound can be produced from serotonin, as shown in Figure 4. Serotonin,

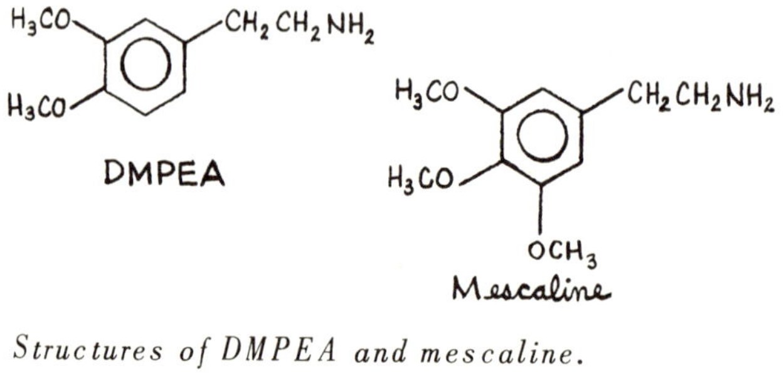

Figure 3: Structures of DMPEA and mescaline.

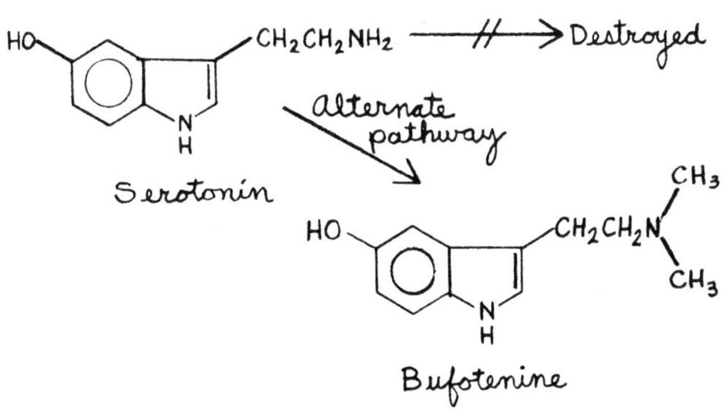

Figure 4: Formation of bufotenine from serotonin.

like norepinephrine, is an intercell chemical communicating agent present in significant amounts in the brain. Normally, serotonin is consumed by a series of biological reactions as soon as it is used. Under
certain conditions the destructive pathway can be blocked, as indicated
in Figure 4. When this happens, serotonin may react by a different
pathway to form bufotenine. Bufotenine, a known hallucinogen, was
first isolated from the skin of toads. It is one of several compounds
which contribute to the renowned poison of these animals. Bufotenine
is almost certainly produced in normal brains, and, perhaps in greater
quantity, in the brains of schizophrenics. Whether or not bufotenine is
actually the intoxicant that produces schizophrenia is not yet known.
This suggestion has only been on the firing line for a few years. Other
hypotheses, such as those concerning adrenochrome and dimethoxyphenethylamine, have been available for 15 or 20 years, which gives
more time for careful work which can prove that they are wrong. While
the bufotenine hypothesis may be just as wrong, this agent remains as
one of the latest in a series of candidates for the role of the elusive
endogeneous hallucinogen. Research over the next few years will
clarify the character of not only bufotenine, but many other components
which have been suggested.

LOOSE ENDS

Although the autointoxication hypothesis has provided the focus
for years of research into schizophrenia, it is not without drawbacks.
Let me point out just one of them. A number of hallucinogenic agents
are now available. Many of these are being tested extensively, either

in scientific laboratories or under less well-controlled conditions. The results of these tests can be correlated. The feeling among many psychiatrists is that the psychotic condition produced by these exogenously administered hallucinogens is not truly the same as that seen in schizophrenia. If we accept this viewpoint, we may be fooling ourselves when we assume that a compound such as bufotenine, known to be an exogenous hallucinogen, may be an intrinsic intoxicating agent. Many psychiatrists insist that there are far more variables involved in autointoxication than are represented by the present data on administered hallucinogens. For example, different dosages produce qualitatively different effects rather than just differences in degree. It is also possible that two compounds present simultaneously may give quite different responses than those seen with either one alone, and so on. On the other hand, some researchers feel that if one increases the dose of any of the hallucinogenic compounds enough, all of them will will produce functionally identical psychoses—strong evidence, if proven, that autointoxication may be the mechanism of schizophrenia. Unfortunately, the conflicting arguments concerning the autointoxication story are voluminous. Autointoxication should be considered simply an hypothesis, to be either accepted or refuted as more evidence becomes available during the next few years.

The chemistry leading to the identification of reserpine and other tranquilizers has given us an effective means of treating schizophrenia. Chemistry has further supplied us a means of looking, however fruit lessly so far, for the causative agents in schizophrenia. A third aspect of the attack on this disease is the search for a simple diagnostic test with which schizophrenia could be located in a population. The problem is not as trivial as it may sound. Over the past hundred years, a large number of different "schizophrenias" have been described. If each of these were truly a different disease, the problem of curing schizophrenia would be difficult indeed. Lately we have begun, however, to believe that only one, or a few, fundamentally different diseases exist, with many variations in their expression. One of the best evidences we have that many varieties of mental illness are manifestations of a single disease is that a number of them respond equally well to treatment with chlorpromazine, suggesting that the fundamental defect in each is similar. If so, all schizophrenics may have some similar alteration in biochemistry which might be detected by the proper analytical techniques.

Although the studies we have considered have not demonstrated the presence of such an identifiable agent, nonetheless, it appears possible that one exists. Beginning hospital personnel are often told that mental wards can be recognized simply by their smell. This odor, long associated with the schizophrenics on the wards, has even been used for diagnostic purposes, using specially trained rats. *Science* magazine in October, 1969, reported a study in which sweat from schizophrenics was examined. The compound responsible for this odor is a *trans*-methylhexenoic acid, a simple seven-carbon compound (Figure 5). It has been found now in the sweat of almost every schizophrenic examined. Although the compound is probably synthesized in the sweat glands, and therefore probably has no causal relationship to schizophrenia (it is difficult to see how the sweat glands could be too influential in controlling the brain), it may well serve as a useful diagnostic tool. Some day it may be possible for a patient to walk into a doctor's office and be subjected to a very simple skin test which can inform the doctor that the man has "chemically diagnosed" schizophrenia, or may have a pre-disposition toward schizophrenia. If the patient is not showing symptoms, it may be possible to treat him in order to prevent any attacks of the disease.

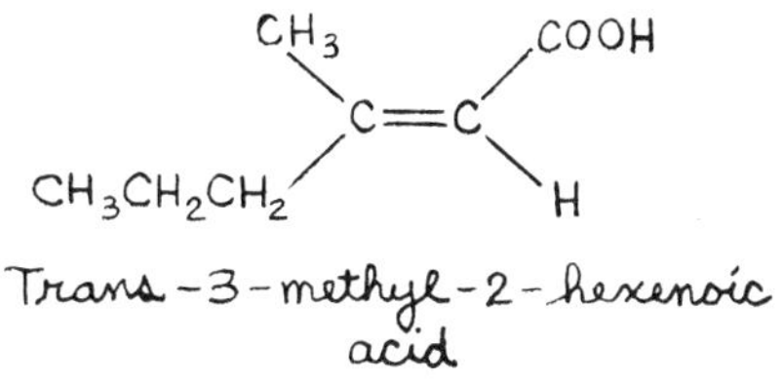

Figure 5: Structure of Trans-3-methyl-2-hexenoic acid.

Such speculation is admittedly going beyond the available data. Nonetheless, the development of diagnostic aids appears to be one direction in which we must move if we are effectively to combat schizophrenia. We can hope that better diagnostic aids, together with ever more effective chemical treatment, will diminish the toll of schizophrenia and will free countless thousands of people now afflicted by this demeaning and unpleasant illness.

SUGGESTED READING.

Kreig, B., Green Medicine, New York, Rand McNally and Co., 1964.
Eiduson, S., Geller, E., Yuwiler, A., and Eiduson, B., Biochemistry and Behavior, New York, Van Nostrand Reinhold, 1964.

IF ANTIBIOTICS ARE SO DAMNED GOOD, WHY AM I STILL SICK?

Kenneth L. Rinehart, Jr.

The question comes from a former coworker in our laboratory, a graduate student with a cold. Under that title I want to discuss antibiotics in general and, especially, what I think is happening with antibiotics research today.

CURRENT CONCERNS OVER ANTIBIOTICS

Over the past few years, and during the past two or three in particular, antibiotics have been getting rather a bad press. When an antibiotic is mentioned in a headline the story is likely to be uncomplimentary. I can illustrate this with a few examples excised from various sources.

One of the places where one can read a good deal about antibiotics is *Biomedical News,* a monthly summary of events in the biomedical community. *Biomedical News* dated August 1970 read "FDA Halts Sale of Multibiotics With Penicillin," Does that imply that penicillin is now bad, whereas it used to be good? Not at all. What the article refers to is a ban on fixed combinations of drugs. Probably the most publicized example of fixed combinations is a drug called Pan-Alba, a drug which the Food and Drug Administration (FDA) asked The Upjohn Company to take off the market. The company resisted in the courts, but the courts held with the FDA, and the drug was removed.

The headline refers, however, not only to Pan-Alba, but to all fixed combinations of antibiotics. Why should the FDA be worried about combinations of antibiotics? The National Academy of Sciences established a committee a few years ago to study whether fixed combinations of drugs, in particular combinations of antibiotics, had been shown to be efficacious beyond the efficacy of the individual drugs. This committee was set up mainly as a result of attacks from a number of quarters on fixed combinations of antibiotics. The reasoning behind the study can be summarized in an article by Ernest Jawetz of the University of California Medical School.

To Dr. Jawetz there were three reasons why fixed combinations of antibiotics cannot be regarded as beneficial. First of all, he says, use of a combination of antibiotics is simply poor medicine, hindering the diagnosis of what is wrong with the patient. This is because the combination of two or more antibiotics in one package is unlikely to be of the optimal ratio to benefit the patient. The rationale, of course, is that if one antibiotic is good, maybe two antibiotics will complement one another and will be better. The optimum procedure would be to take a culture of the disease-causing organism, find out which antibiotic will kill that organism most efficiently, and then use that antibiotic. However, if one doesn't have the time or the facilities for doing these culture determinations, it is tempting to use a "shotgun" approach, giving a large number of antibiotics, the sum of which may prove efficacious. This could discourage diagnosis, providing a false sense of security to both the physician and the patient, and inevitably the dosage must be wrong because there is an optimum antibiotic and an optimum dose for every infection.

Second, many antibiotics are toxic, others cause hypersensitivity and allergic reactions. Dr. Jawetz reasons that a combination of antibiotics enhances the direct toxic effects of each: Although two antibiotics may have more chance of killing an organism, they also have more chance of causing toxic reactions and hypersensitivity. Penicillin is of course a prime offender, as a large portion of the population is sensitive to penicillin.

Third, combination therapy may favor the emergence of resistant strains of organisms which previously were killed by an antibiotic. By using a shotgun approach, employing two, three, or four antibiotics, the organism may become resistant to two, three, or four, rather than just one.

Let us turn now to other headlines, taken from *Biomedical News* and the *New York Times*. These read: "FDA Looking at Antibiotics in Feed;" "FDA to Act on Animal Feeds;" and "U.S. Moving to Sue Farmers for Trace of Drugs in Cattle." So what is wrong with antibiotics in feeds? This problem, too, has been studied by a committee, a task force of the Food and Drug Administration, which made its report in 1970. One of my colleagues at the University of Illinois, William Huber, a pharmacologist in the College of Veterinary Medicine, was a member of that task force and has written extensively on the subject, in this book[1] and elsewhere.

The problem is that antibiotics in feeds sometimes turn up in meat, and Huber cites very interesting statistics ascertained by his group at the University of Illinois. Although antibiotics are, in fact, banned from meat, although there is a law which says that antibiotics may not appear in meat, Huber's group found a surprisingly high percentage of meat does contain antibiotic residues.

How do antibiotics get in meat? The answer in simple enough. Over one-half of the antibiotics that are produced in the U.S. go into agricultural products, rather than into human therapy. Of course, all the feed supplements indicate the withdrawal time required before slaughtering, but apparently some people either do not read the instructions or simply ignore them.

If there are antibiotics in meat and we know why they are there, is their presence a bad thing? Potentially, at least, it is. As pointed out before in this chapter, some antibiotics are toxic, giving serious toxic symptoms, especially when injected into the blood stream. Other antibiotics cause sensitization of humans.

Another apprehension arising from the use of antibiotics in feed and feed supplements is that they will induce resistance in the organisms which inhabit the animals and that the resistant organisms, perhaps pathogenic, may then either be transmitted directly to people or that they may transfer their resistance to antibiotics to other microorganisms by a molecular mechanism of resistance transfer. These concerns are described in greater detail in Dr. Huber's chapter.

Let us turn to other headlines, one in *Biomedical News* for February 1971: "Hospital Infection on the Increase," one in the February 3, 1971 *Wall Street Journal*, "Stubborn Germs: Increasing Resistance of Bacteria to Drugs Causes New Concern." Infection has been an increasing problem in hospitals during the past few years. Resistant strains of infecting organisms tend to arise in hospitals because of the organisms' exposure to antibiotics there. Worse, as people return from hospitals to their community they spread these resistant organisms to a wider circle of people than is exposed in hospitals. Moreover, antibiotics in food, cosmetics, and hygienic products change the normal microbial flora that one has constantly on his skin and in his intestines in subtle ways. These organisms may then become resistant to antibiotics. In hospitals, the problem tends to be centered on severe

---

[1]See W. G. Huber, "The Meat We Eat," in this book.

gram-negative infections, especially *Pseudomonas* infections, which have doubled in frequency the last five years. These infections occur after surgery or severe burns, and they also provide complications in the treatment of leukemia, cystic fibrosis, and other diseases unrelated to the *Pseudomonas* infection.

By now two recurring themes are apparent: the sensitization of an individual to antibiotics, and the development of resistant strains of microorganisms.

THE GOLDEN ERA OF ANTIBIOTICS

These headlines on antibiotics in recent times contrast rather markedly with what might be called the golden days or golden era of antibiotics. In that era, lasting roughly from about 1943 to 1960, antibiotics were generally regarded as true wonder drugs. It is probably difficult for most of us to remember the days before 1940 - before World War II. These were days in which bacterial infectious diseases were one of the prime causes of death in this country and throughout the world. I grew up an only child because my sister died in 1927 of pneumonia, in those days a very common cause of death among infants. Pneumonia is rarely fatal now among the otherwise healthy, and infectious diseases in general are no longer a common cause of death.

During World War II penicillin was developed, primarily for the military forces to cure staphylococcus infections in wounds. When it was introduced immediately after the war to the civilian market, one had the feeling that infectious diseases were licked, that there was no longer going to be any problem with bacteria at all. The story generally went around in those days that it was cheaper to get rid of gonorrhea than to get it, that one shot of penicillin would cure it. Those were the days in which Nobel prizes were awarded for antibiotics research--to Alexander Fleming, Howard Florey, and E. B. Chain, who worked at Oxford, and to Selman Waksman at the Rutgers Institute of Microbiology. These were the biologists who discovered penicillin, streptomycin, neomycin, and actinomycin, famous antibiotics still in use. The antibiotics also proved of great interest to chemists because many of the compounds had remarkable structures of types never seen before, either in nature or in test tubes. At least three chemists who have received recent Nobel Prizes, Robert Woodward, Lord Todd, and Derek Barton, have worked in part with these complex compounds.

Those were indeed golden days and antibiotics in the context of pre-World War II medicine were wonder drugs. Moreover, if antibiotics have encountered problems, most of the difficulties are really the price of success. Antibiotics have simply been too good. Relatively few people die today of infectious diseases. The death rate from staphylococcal pneumonia prior to the introduction of antibiotics was 35 per cent, today it is about 15 per cent. The death rate from staphylococcal septicemia before antibiotics was 90 per cent, now it is about 25 per cent. Antibiotics do save lives.

A small book called "*The Life Sciences*" was published by the National Academy of Sciences about two years ago. In a section dealing with antibiotics the book makes the following statement: "Although there is as yet no universally effective agent, one or another of these drugs, antibiotics, can mitigate virtually all known infections. Antibiotics have drastically altered the patterns of medical practice. Prior to 1940 thousands of hospital beds were occupied by patients with infectious diseases. Today, in the main, these patients receive a prescription for antibiotics and return home. The morbidity associated with postoperative infections has dropped sharply. The damaging, once frequent, chain of events that began with a strep throat and went on to scarlet fever, rheumatic fever and serious heart disease has been broken."

I think most parents are used to calling the pediatrician, describing the symptoms on the telephone, and having the pediatrician call in a prescription to the drug store. And in nearly every case the child recovers very quickly.

Antibiotics are the treatment of choice in nearly all microbial infections. The October 4, 1968, **Medical Letter** listed 67 infectious organisms that the physician is likely to encounter. For the treatment of infections caused by those 67 organisms there were only five drugs listed which were not antibiotics. The drugs of first choice were nearly all antibiotics. Penicillin was the first choice for the largest number of organisms, followed by tetracycline, amphotericin B, ampicillin, a newer version of penicillin, streptomycin, erythromycin, and kanamycin.

The Medical Letter also gave a list of alternative drugs, the second choices. On that list tetracycline led, followed by erythromycin, chloramphenicol, and streptomycin. On this list of alternatives some of the compounds tend to be rather toxic. In particular, chloramphenicol has some very serious anemia-causing problems and it is used only where there is a serious infection.

Now we should examine the dates when those drugs were introduced or discovered. Going down the list in order of frequency as antibiotic of first choice one finds: penicillin, introduced in 1940; tetracycline, 1948; amphotericin B, 1956; ampicillin, 1965; streptomycin, 1944; erythromycin, 1952; kanamycin, 1957. Except for ampicillin, which is a modified penicillin, these are all relatively old antibiotics. It appears that new antibiotics are not being introduced very rapidly.

SOURCES OF ANTIBIOTICS

Just what are antibiotics? How are they obtained? Where do they come from? The most widely accepted definition is that of Selman Waksman, coined perhaps 30 years ago. Waksman's definition is that "An antibiotic is a chemical substance produced by microorganisms, which in very low concentration has the capacity to inhibit the growth and even to destroy bacteria and other microorganisms."

There really are four parts to that definition. First, an antibiotic kills microorganisms—infectious organisms or others, beneficial organisms as well as harmful. Second, although many compounds are active against microorganisms, not very many are active in minute concentrations. Third, an antibiotic is a chemical substance and a chemist should be able to deduce the structure of the compound—perhaps synthesize it, perhaps try to figure out how it is made in nature. Fourth, an antibiotic must be produced by a microorganism. Compounds from many sources kill microorganisms, but, in order to be an antibiotic by Waksman's generally-accepted definition, the compound has to be pro-produced by another microorganism.

A few fungi produce antibiotics, the most notable being *Penicillium notatum*, which produces penicillin, but not very many fungi produce good antibiotics. A few bacteria yield antibiotics, including the commercially available bacitracin, gramicidin, and polymyxin, but not many bacteria produce antibiotics. Nearly all of the antibiotics which are used in medicine today come from actinomycetes (mainly the genus *Streptomyces*), which are neither fungi nor bacteria but lie somewhere between the two on the taxonomic scale.

How do scientists find new antibiotics? Since they are produced by microorganisms, one goes to any place where microorganisms are found, especially to the soil. To quote Selman Waksman again (and the Bible), "From the earth shall come thy salvation." Soil has enormous numbers of microorganisms, so initially one begins by collecting soil samples more or less at random around the world. That is how most antibiotics were found. A soil sample from Venezuela gave us *Streptomyces venezuelae*, which produces chloramphenicol, but a soil sample collected in a backyard in New Haven, Conn., gave the same microorganism and the same antibiotic. Thus, antibiotics can come from exotic places or they can come from our own backyards. Very often one finds the same antibiotic being produced from soil samples isolated in many different parts of the world.

Soil samples are collected and sent to a microbiologist, who then ascertains whether a particular soil sample has microorganisms living in it that produce active antibiotics. He does this by trying to culture the organisms growing in the soil. This involves suspending the soil sample in water and diluting the suspension enormously, then transferring drops of the diluted suspension to a mixture of nutrients to see what grows. These organisms are usually actinomycetes and they grow in spore colonies, as shown in the picture. Small colonies of these spores are then transferred to shake flasks containing nutrient medium.

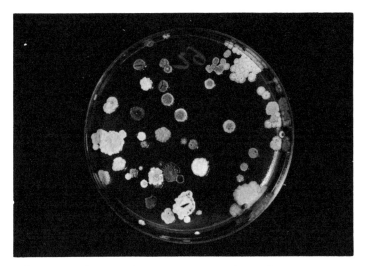

Figure 1: Colonies of several organisms, mostly actinomycetes, growing in a Petri dish. (Courtesy of The Upjohn Company, Kalamazoo, Mich.)

When the organism grows it is tested for antibiotic production by adding an extract to filter paper disks which are placed on an agar plate containing a test organism, for example *Bacillus subtilus* or *Escherichia coli*, which can be killed by an antibiotic. The test organism growing on the plate makes it rather opaque, but there may be clear areas in which the bacterium is inhibited from growing, as shown in the picture. If this occurs, it indicates the presence of an antibiotic.

If an antibiotic is present, it must be identified. After the organism has been grown it is filtered off and extracted to obtain the antibiotic, whether it is in the filtrate or extract. A two-fold approach then

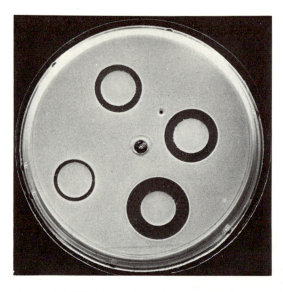

Figure 2: The rings of inhibition show the action of an antibiotic at different concentrations against the bacterium "Bacillus subtilis" on a nutrient agar medium. (Courtesy of The Upjohn Company, Kalamazoo, Mich.)

begins—involving attempts to identify both the microorganism and the antibiotic it produces. The identification of the microorganism involves microbiologists, the identification of the antibiotic involves chemists and biochemists. At this point the antibiotic is terribly impure, so any method for identifying it requires doing so in an impure state. The most useful approach is an antimicrobial spectrum, which is a table of all the bacteria and other organisms that the antibiotic kills. Not all antibiotics kill all organisms, as shown in the picture, and one can often get an insight into the nature of the antibiotic—what kind of compound one is dealing with—from this antimicrobial spectrum. An additional help in identification is a paper chromatogram, with which one can see how fast the antibiotic moves in a solvent system up the strip of paper. To find the antibiotic the paper chromatogram is overlaid with an agar strip containing a test organism which is inhibited by the antibiotic. Different antibiotics move at different rates and one can often tell pretty well what sort of antibiotic he is dealing with by this characteristic. It may be a known compound.

   If it is a known antibiotic, then the whole subject is usually dropped, because it is neither fun nor profitable doing the same research over again. On the other hand, if the antibiotic is a new compound and its antimicrobial spectrum is interesting, the scale is increased for a pilot run in a tank of perhaps 250-gallon volume, which will produce enough of the material to isolate and identify chemically.

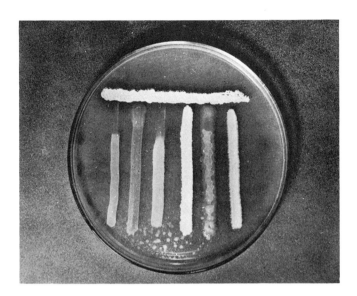

Figure 3: On this agar plate six streaks of various kinds of bacteria are shown at right angles to a streak of an antibiotic-producing organism. Four of the bacteria are sensitive to the antibiotic and have disappeared near the antibiotic source; two are resistant to the antibiotic. (Courtesy of Eli Lilly and Company, Indianapolis, Ind.)

The purification of the material obtained from the tank is followed by much the same procedure of bioassay. Ultimately, the pure compound in hand, one attempts to find out what its structure is. While the isolation and structure work are going on, the microbiologists are working, too. They perform *in vitro* studies first to see just how much of the compound is required to kill different organisms, establishing a quantitative antimicrobial spectrum. If that shows the compound to be a useful antibiotic, then they go on to *in vivo* studies in animals—mice, dogs, and perhaps monkeys. These studies continue as long as two criteria are satisfied: the antibiotic has to be a new compound, and it also has to be both efficacious in getting rid of infecting organisms and safe in the animals. Finally, one might to on to clinical trials after filing a plan for the clinical trial with the Food and Drug Administration. A clinical trial again would establish, this time in humans, whether the new antibiotic is effective and whether it is safe. At this stage a decision must be reached as to whether the new compound is better than present antibiotics that do much the same thing. If it is better than those presently available, it is marketed and one day we see it appearing on physicians' prescription lists and on pharmacists' shelves. Only if it is efficacious and safe, it is approved by the Food and Drug Administration.

REDUCTION IN ANTIBIOTICS RESEARCH

In the earlier section where we discussed the **Medical Letter's** antibiotics of choice in the treatment of infectious diseases, we noted that most are *old* antibiotics. This point has also been made by Lloyd Conover of Pfizer Laboratories in his chapter of a recent book entitled "Drug Discovery". Dr. Conover noted that the rate at which new antibiotics have been introduced to the market has in fact fallen off very sharply; from a peak in the five-year period 1955 to 1959, the number introduced between 1960 and 1964 decreased, and in the period 1965 to 1969, there weren't any new antibiotics.

One reason for the reduction in the numbers of antibiotics being introduced has to do with problems in marketing a new antibiotic. These are basically two-fold: the new antibiotic must be superior to an old compound, and it must be approved by the Food and Drug Administration. The latter process, especially, is exceedingly expensive and takes a very long time.[2] Of the thousands or so antibiotics which have been discovered over the years, there are probably fewer than 40 that have ever been marketed.

Another reason fewer antibiotics are being introduced, according to Conover, is that a number of people have concluded that the classical antibiotic screening process (The process starting with soil samples described above) is relatively futile. Conover sent out questionnaires to scientists engaged in antibiotics research and on the basis of returns from the questionnaire came to his conclusion. He argues that the time for screening is probably over and a number of pharmaceutical companies apparently agree, since they have quit screening for antibiotics. Those which continue to screen do so on a much smaller scale than before.

Although Conover concluded that the old screening procedure is unproductive, he suggested in his questionnaire a number of possible ways of looking for new antibiotics, which his respondents voted on. The favored approach among the respondents in his poll was continued screening but with different procedures. First was the possibility of applying new techniques for the collection, storage, and processing of soil samples. For example, rather than using the usual nutrient media, one might try new media to get different organisms to grow from the old soil samples. One might also do a better job of detecting antibiotics when are there. The possibility voted second was the examination of new genera of microorganisms. Until now, **Streptomycetes** have been

---

[2]Though probably not as long as the process involved in marketing a new birth control drug; see Carl Djerassi, "Birth Control after 1984," in this book.

mainly looked at, but rather recently other genera have been examined. For example, the *Micromonospora* have produced a very successful antibiotic called gentamicin. In third place was the potentiality of examining marine microorganisms. This possibility—antibiotics from the sea—has attracted considerable newspaper attention. In fourth place was the examination of terrestrial microorganisms that grow under unusual or extreme environmental conditions—for example, an organism growing in the Great Salt Lake may produce something different from organisms growing in soil. Finally, examination of microorganisms that grow in the presence of pathogens might produce new antibiotics. These five possibilities have not been exhausted and they are all being investigated.

Other approaches to developing new antibiotics, which do not involve screening organisms, were also suggested. The preparation of structural analogs of useful antibiotics by chemical or other means was regarded as especially promising. This involves modifying an old antibiotic by one means or another to make a new antibiotic. Chemical modification has accounted for more new antibiotics in recent years than screening. A final possibility suggested by Conover was the preparation of structural analogs of compounds that have been rejected in the past because they were toxic or because they were poorly efficacious.

Still another reason that new antibiotics are not being introduced is that antibiotics are cures for infectious diseases, while both the biomedical community and federal government funding have shifted their attention from infectious diseases to cancer and heart disease. Harold Schmeck reported in the *New York Times* for February 10, 1973 that influenza and pneumonia together rank first among diseases in terms of disability days and upper respiratory diseases rank second. Similarly, *Biomedical News* for August 1972 noted in an interview with Dr. Dorland Davis that over half of patients' visits to physicians are related to infections and respiratory ailments. Yet the National Institute of Allergy and Infectious Diseases (NIAID), which Dr. Davis heads, ranks seventh among the 11 major units of the National Institutes of Health (NIH) in terms of budget appropriations. Since NIAID sponsors research on allergy and infectious diseases in universities and medical schools and its budget has remained static in recent years, the implications for antibiotics research are clear. Even within NIAID the emphasis in research on infectious diseases has shifted away from antibiotics and toward immunology. In a talk presented by Dr. Davis before the Infectious Diseases Society of America he listed eight special emphasis programs of NIAID for research on infectious diseases. In only two of these were antibiotics mentioned: the drug resistance program included a continued search for antibiotics to use against drug-resistant bacteria and meningococci, and the antiviral substances program included study of the mechanism of action of antibiotics on viral replication. This relative lack of emphasis on the part of funding agencies assures that less research will be carried out on antibiotics today than a few years ago and is another reason not many new antibiotics are being developed.

THE FUTURE OF ANTIBIOTICS RESEARCH

Although both Dr. Davis at the NIH and Dr. Conover at Pfizer are somewhat pessimistic, work on antibiotics does continue. What are the current research areas where people are working today on antibiotics? First, chemists are correlating the structures of known antibiotics. When antibiotics were first isolated it seemed that the structure of every new antibiotic represented a unique structural type. Now that over a thousand antibiotics have been isolated and over a hundred structures have been established, we know that their structures allow the compounds to be divided into classes of antibiotics. They can be arranged in various ways, but I prefer to divide them according to where their atoms come from biosynthetically.

Antibiotics of acetate or propionate origin (related, distantly, to fatty acids) include polyene antibiotics like amphotericin B, which are antifungal agents, macrolide antibiotics like erythromycin, aromatic antibiotics like the tetracyclines, and ansamycin antibiotics like rifampicin. A second class contains the peptide antibiotics, which include bacitracin, polymyxin, and actinomycin, together with those derived from peptides, like penicillin and cephalosporin. Some antibiotics are carbohydratelike. These include neomycin, streptomycin, and lincomycin, which are all well known. Finally, a few antibiotics are related to nucleosides; these tend to be antitumor agents, like puromycin.

A second active area of investigation is chemical synthesis. From a knowledge of the structures of antibiotics and the activity correlations that can be derived from these structures it is often possible to predict the structure of a new active antibiotic. This knowledge keeps chemists active synthesizing new antibiotics related to old ones—with some success, as noted by Dr. Conover. Under successful chemically synthesized antibiotics we can list the cephalosporins and newer penicillins, largely made by semi-synthetic procedures, and clindamycin, a new antibiotic related to lincomycin.

A third area of antibiotics research in which people are working very hard these days is biosynthesis. If one looks at the structure of an antibiotic he can guess what sort of things might go into producing that antibiotic in nature. For example, as soon as the structure of

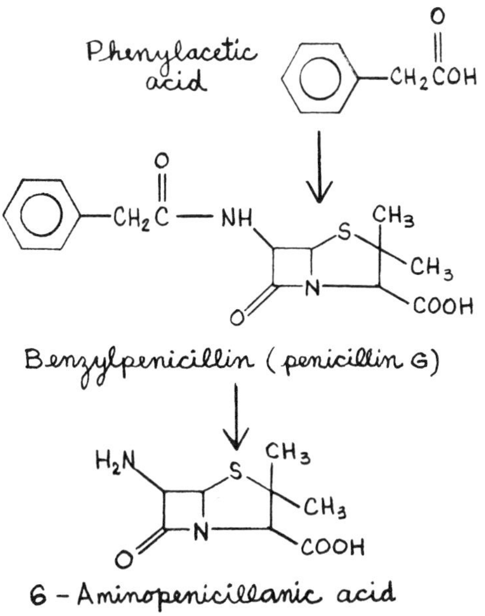

Figure 4: The subunits of benzylpenicillin.

pencillin was established, around 1945, it became clear that it must be derived from phenylacetic acid. Biochemists then began adding phenylacetic acid to the penicillin fermentation medium, according to the scheme in Figure 4, and immediately the production of penicillin jumped by a factor of about 20. Going a step further, it was argued that it might be possible to alter the fermentation conditions so that one would get just a piece of the penicillin molecule, on which one could put other groups. Thus, 6-aminopenicillanic acid is now prepared by fermentation and one can tack on to it other acyl groups instead of phenylacetyl. This is the origin of the semisynthetic penicillins like ampicillin, one of the common antibiotics of choice. In our own laboratory we have been utilizing a somewhat different procedure in altering antibiotic biosynthesis. We tried to find out first what the biosynthetic pathway of neomycin was, then we attempted to mutate the organism so that it could no longer make one of the subunits of neomycin. Then we added other compounds to the fermentation media to replace that subunit and make new antibiotics, which we call hybrimycins.

A fourth exciting area of investigation of antibiotics involves determining the mechanism of resistance by other organisms. For example, we know that many of the organisms which initially were killed by penicillin have through the years become resistant to that antibiotic. It was initially thought that the development of resistance was mainly a matter of bacterial mutation. According to this mechanism bacteria, in the presence of an antibiotic, occasionally mutate spontaneously and one of these mutations may make them resistant to the antibiotic. Since the mutations should be random, one of the desired sort (from the bacteria's standpoint) should not happen very often, making this a rather reassuring hypothesis (from the human's standpoint). Apparently such mutation does happen. In the case of penicillin-resistant organisms, mutation has developed organisms which produce an enzyme called penicillinase, which hydrolyzes penicillin to an inactive material. Penicillinase has been isolated and can be used in testing a new penicillin for activity against penicillin-resistant organisms, by seeing whether it is cleaved by penicillinase rather than testing it against the organism itself. This has some clear advantages for the chemist. It is assumed in the mutation hypothesis that resistance is a part of the genetic material which is simply transferred from one generation of a bacterium to the next.

More recently, a second, far more frightening mechanism of resistance development has emerged. This, the socalled resistance transfer factor or R-factor, is what the *Wall Street Journal* article was referring to. The R-factor seems to be a type of DNA not associated with the chromosomes of the bacteria but which can actually be transferred from one cell to another and even from one organism to a different organism, via the mechanism of conjugation. And these organisms don't necessarily have to be very closely related. Relatively harmless bacteria

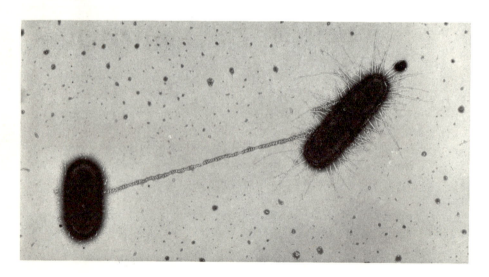

Figure 5: Resistance transfer factor (RTF) is thought to be transferred from one bacterial cell to another through conjugation by way of thin tubules called pili. (From an electron micrograph made by Charles C. Brinton, Jr., and Judith Carnahan, University of Pittsburgh.)

like E. *coli* can transfer their resistance to neomycin or streptomycin to pathogenic organisms like **Klebsiella pneumoniae** by actual injection or transfer of this R-factor, which is apparently a cyclic DNA.

Study of the mechanism of resistance development or mechanism of inactivation can prove fruitful in designing antibiotics. For example, there are at least two different ways that kanamycin, a very effective antibiotic, can be inactivated (Figure 6). One way is by the acetylation of an amino group in the 6-position of one of its components. The other way is by the phosphorylation of a hydroxyl group in the 2-position

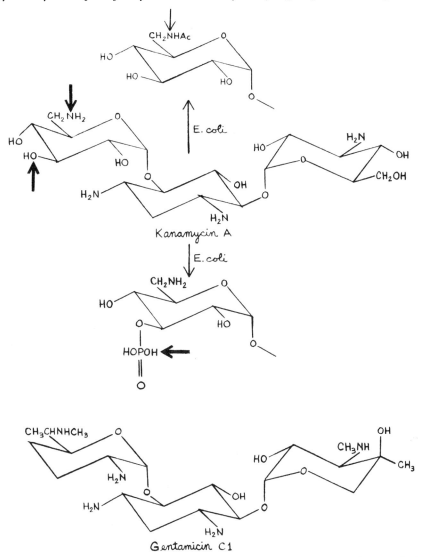

Figure 6: Inactivation of kanamycin by phosphorylation and acetylation.

of that same component. Knowing this, one can make new and better kanamycins which don't have the hydroxyl group in the 2-position for phosphorylation, or which don't have the amino group in the 6-position for acetylation. New kanamycins of this sort, which are not inactivated by resistant bacteria, have been prepared. It also appears to be no accident that a related antibiotic called gentamicin, which is replacing kanamycin, just happens to lack the 2-hydroxyl and 6-amino groups.

The fifth and last area of active investigation is the mode of action of antibiotics. This is essentially the opposite of resistance development, as it is the mechanism by which the antibiotic actually succeeds in killing a microorganism. Study of mode of action has led to some very interesting recent developments. There are relatively few known modes of action. Perhaps the oldest recognized mechanism is interference with a growth factor. For example sulfanilamide looks structurally like *para*-aminobenzoic acid, a growth factor for bacteria. Sulfanilamide can replace the natural compound in early stages of metabolism but then clogs the metabolic pathway and kills the organism. The sulfa drugs work this way but most antibiotics work by different methods.

Penicillin works by inhibiting cell wall synthesis of the bacteria. Since the cell walls protect the bacteria from the environment, prevention of cell wall synthesis kills the bacteria. Other antibiotics, notably the carbohydrate antibiotics of the streptomycin-neomycin class, function by attaching themselves to the ribosomes of the bacteria. By so doing they confuse protein synthesis, as the ribosomes provide the code for protein synthesis. If the organism therefore synthesizes the wrong proteins or nonsense proteins it is prevented from growing.

Other antibiotics actually prevent protein synthesis in one of several different ways, as shown in Figure 7. One whole class of antibiotics inhibits DNA synthesis; these are largely compounds which have been used as anti-tumor agents. Of course, if no DNA is formed, no RNA can be formed, and if no RNA is formed, protein synthesis is impossible. However, the antibiotic functions by attaching itself to DNA. Humans contain DNA, too, so these antibiotics tend to be rather toxic. Another class of antibiotics inhibits RNA synthesis directly. There are two different mechanisms for the inhibition of RNA synthesis. One class of antibiotics, exemplified by actinomycin, prevents RNA synthesis by attaching itself to the DNA template. Another class inhibits RNA synthesis by reacting with the polymerase which is making the RNA. A final mode of antibiotic action involves inhibition of oxidative phosphorylation, but this is a less important category.

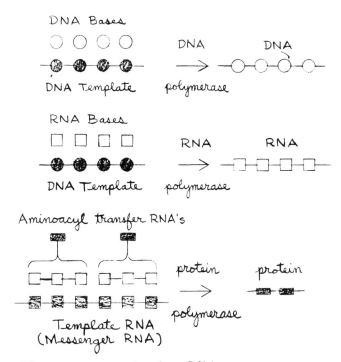

Figure 7: The route to proteins from DNA.

To show how these mode of action studies have proved useful, I shall give a few examples. The polyene antibiotics, in general, have always been regarded as being very active antifugal agents. Amphotericin B was the reagent of choice listed for eight different infectious organisms, all fungi. Nearly all fungal infections are treated by polyene antibiotics. The mode of action of polyene antibiotics involves attack on the cell walls of the fungi. In effect the polyene antibiotics form complexes with steroids found in the cell walls and pull them out of the cell walls leaving holes, so that the protoplasm simply leaks out and the fungus dies. An understanding of this mode of action has led serendipitously to completely new uses for these antibiotics.

A small New York pharmaceutical company was investigating candicidin, a polyene antibiotic like amphotericin B, as an antifungal agent and was testing it on dogs. One rather old dog had a severely enlarged prostate which interfered seriously with urination and sexual activity. However, during treatment with candicidin his prostatitis diminished considerably and he regained his interest in fire hydrants and bitches. This behavior puzzled the veterinarians and they conculted a biochemist as to why this might be. The biochemist reasoned

that since polyenes form complexes with steroids, and since the prostate is associated with male steroidal hormones, that candicidin must
somehow be removing steroids from the system. They then looked at the
blood-cholesterol level of the old dog and found that it had been reduced. At the moment polyene antibiotics are undergoing clinical testing in humans and appear to be promising agents for treating chronic
prostatitis, which afflicts about two-thirds of men over 65, and potential agents for lowering blood-cholesterol levels.

A second example of how an understanding of the mode of action
of an antibiotic can lead to new and interesting drug applications is
the case of the ansa macrolide antibiotics, especially rifampicin. It
has been known for some years that rifampicin is an effective antibacterial agent. Studies have indicated its mode of action involves
inhibition of the DNA-dependent RNA polymerase, the polymerase
which catalyzes the polymerization of nucleosides on a DNA template
to give RNA. About two years ago two groups—those of Howard Temin
at Wisconsin and of David Baltimore at MIT—isolated a new enzyme,
socalled reverse transcriptase, from RNA viruses. Under catalysis of
reverse transcriptase nucleosides are polymerized on an RNA template
to form DNA. This polymerization, the reverse of the usual process,
was proposed as a possible explanation of how RNA viruses can invade
the host organism. Moreover, since leukemia viruses are RNA viruses
this seemed to provide a rational, molecular explanation for the pro-
liferation of some cancers. If one could find a drug which would prevent
the reverse transcriptase catalysis—the RNA-dependent DNA polymerase activity—perhaps one could kill the virus or tumor selectively
without killing the host. On the basis of its activity as an inhibitor
of DNA-dependent RNA polymerase, rifampicin was tested on reverse
transcriptase. In fact, rifampicin is *very* active in inhibiting reverse
transcriptase. Moreover, one of the other ansa macrolide antibiotics,
streptovaricin, has the same activity and has been shown to cause a
reduction of leukemia in mice. From this example we see that knowledge of their mode of action can be a useful tool for predicting what
particular antibiotics might be good for in addition to their antimicrobial roles.

Finally, if one looks into a crystal ball for the future of antibiotics, one sees a number of applications. First, the chief use of
antibiotics in the future will probably continue to be as antibacterial
agents. This is because they are so remarkably good. Within that field
new antibiotics will probably be introduced mainly against resistant
strains—to assist the presently ineffective antibiotics. This is already
the case with ampicillin, the new penicillin effective against resistant

strains of staphylococci. Antibiotics will also be introduced for specific purposes, against specific diseases. A new antibiotic, spection-
mycin, marketed under the trade name of Trobicin, has been introduced
within the last year with really excellent acceptance, for only one
disease: gonorrhea. If the disease is sufficiently widespread, antibiotics can be developed for it.

Antibiotics will also be developed for treatment of fungal infec.
tions; we hope some will be useful for systemic fungal infections.
Some antibiotics will be useful as antiprotozoal agents—as anti-malarial
drugs, for example. We hope that some antibiotics will be useful as
antiviral and antitumor agents. In developing these new applications,
the more we know about the mode of action of antibiotics, the more
successful we will be.

In conclusion, it seems clear that we are still basking in the
twilight of the golden days of exponential growth of antibiotics. However, the golden age was based on a shotgun research approach, with
rather little understanding of the basic science involved. Although the
present reputation of antibiotics is by no means spotless, their future
is far from bleak. It surely will be more difficult to find new antibiotics
—and they will need to be more selective; but the fundamental chemical
and biological knowledge is rapidly accumulating which should allow
us to apply antibiotics not only to the classical field of bacterial infection, but to other disorders and diseases as well.

SUGGESTED READING

Jones, R. G., Antibiotics of the Penicillin and Cephalosporin Family, American Scientist, 58:404, 1970.

Jawetz, E., The Use of Combinations of Antimicrobial Drugs, Ann. Rev. Pharmacol., 8:151, 1968.

Conover, L. H., Discovery of Drugs from Microbiological Sources, *in* Drug Discovery, Science and Development in a Changing Society, Advances in Chemistry Series 108, Washington, D. C., American Chemical Society, 1971, Chap. 3.

Watanabe, T., Infectious Drug Resistance, Scientific American, 217:19, 1967.

Temin, H. M., RNA-Directed DNA Synthesis, Scientific American, 226:24, 1972.

"The Life Sciences," Washington, D. C., National Academy of Sciences, 1970.

Davis, D. J., Remarks on Special Emphasis Programs of the National Institute of Allergy and Infectious Diseases, J. Infectious Diseases, 121:231, 1970.

BIRTH CONTROL PROSPECTS AFTER 1984

Carl Djerassi

The reason birth control is relevant in chemistry is that, in my opinion, most of the future advances in contraception will probably be chemical in nature. It is for this reason that I think that today's topic is really very germane to your series.

The reason for the title "Birth Control After 1984" is twofold. First, I would like to emphasize right at the beginning that the prospects for coming up soon with fundamentally new birth control methods are fairly poor, and that we shall have to wait at least until the 1980's before we can expect them to be available for public consumption. Second, the Orwellian overtones are justified, because I will discuss in part the hypothetical case of a birth control agent that involves addition to food and water—a concept which would clearly fall within the definition of an Orwellian society.

I shall go quickly through some nonchemical material which will tell you why the topic that I am discussing is of crucial importance and why a solution to the problem is so urgent. Figure 1 shows the growth of the world's population since the birth of Christ. You will note that it took 1800 years to reach the first billion, 100 years to reach the second billion, 30 years to the third billion and only 15 years to the fourth billion. The dotted lines show the extrapolation for the rest of this century. As you see, it will probably take only nine years to come up with the next billion people on this earth.

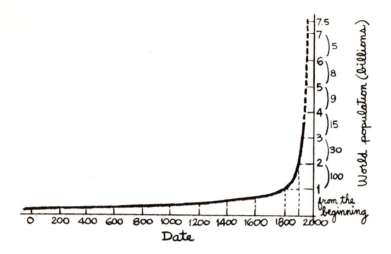

Figure 1: From P. Handler, "Biology and the Future of Man," New York, Oxford University Press, 1970.

In Table 1 you will see the problem expressed in a different way, by the number of years it took to double the world's population. It took well over 1500 years to double it the first time around, using the birth of Christ again as the reference point. It took 200 years to increase it from half a billion to one billion. By extrapolating from 1975 onward, it will take only about 30 years to double the world's population unless something dramatic is done quickly, which is very unlikely. The most likely extrapolation indicates that we will have somewhere between seven and one-half to eight billion people by the turn of the century, compared to about three and one-half billion right now.

TABLE 1
Time required to double world population.

World Population	Year	Time Required
250,000,000	1	
		1649
500,000,000	1650	
		200
1,000,000,000	1850	
		80
2,000,000,000	1930	
		45[1]
4,000,000,000	1975[1]	
		30[1]
8,000,000,000	2005[1]	

[1]Estimate.

I need also to refer to one other magic figure, the per cent population increase each year. You hear that western European countries and the United States have an annual percentage population increase of something on the order of 1 or 1.5 per cent. This appears to be piddling. You wouldn't want to put your money in a bank and just get one and half per cent per year interest. And yet, such a percentage return corresponds to a doubling every 70 years or so. In the context of the world's population, starting with three billion (which is what we had fairly recently) would mean that we would be at the level of 6 billion in 70 years. If we reached a 3 per cent growth per year, which still appears to be a very small figure, the world's population would double every 23 years. At 4 per cent, it would double every 17 years. The consequences of these figures are quite fantastic and I shall leave them to your imagination.

The annual population growths of most Latin American countries are in the 3 to 3.5 per cent class. There are a few exceptions—Argentina and Uruguay—which are in the European range of 1 or 1.5 per cent. This means that most of the countries in Latin America will double their population about every 20 years. To put it in the context of a neighboring country, the population of Mexico may reach 80 million in the 1980's. The reason I picked Latin America—I could show you equally gruesome figures from many other countries—is that the question of religion, particularly the position of the Catholic Church, comes in at a very early stage when one discusses birth control. There is one common denominator about Latin America—it is well over 90 per cent Catholic. Argentina and Uruguay are as Catholic as Brazil and Chile and yet you see that Argentina and Uruguay have birth rates that are very similar to those of western Europe, while the rest of the Latin American countries have very high birth rates. Furthermore, Chile, a country located geographically rather close to Brazil, has an active and large government-sponsored birth control program, whereas Brazil currently opposes such programs as a matter of government policy.

One of the consequences of such very rapid population growth rates is illustrated in Table 2, with Costa Rica, which has, perhaps, the highest birth rate in Latin America; and Denmark, which has a typically low western European birth rate. One of the very important

TABLE 2
Age distribution as percentage of population (1963).

	Under 15 Years	15 - 40 Years	Over 40 Years
Costa Rica	48%	34%	18%
Denmark	24%	35%	41%

consequences is the age distribution of the population. Specifically, you find nearly half the people in Costa Rica under the age of 15, whereas only 24 per cent fall in that age group in Denmark. On the other hand, people over the age of 40 years make up 40 per cent of the Danish population, but only 18 per cent of that in Costa Rica. The American situation is rather similar to that of Denmark. I don't think I need to go into the further consequences of this skewed age distribution other than to point out, for example, that Costa Rica adds in any one year an abnormally large number of people to the new labor pool. This is particularly bad for economies which cannot absorb or employ all the people they already have in their existing labor pool, let alone all the new ones added each year.

Latin America will show a major increase in population by the year 2000, but in comparison to those of India and China, it will be relatively small. Population projections to the year 2000 become particularly significant in the context of Table 3, which really defines the crux of the population explosion—two words which are usually meant to refer to the explosion in numbers. I intend to use these words in a different context. I refer to the geopolitical explosion which will certainly occur if the population growth is not checked very rapidly. Table 3 offers a stark comparison between North America and Asia, which occupy approximately the same proportion, 16 and 18 per cent, respectively, of the world's land surface. North America contains only about 10 per cent of the world's population whereas Asia has over half of the world's population. And yet, the 10 per cent that live in North America own nearly half the world's wealth, while that half of the world's population living in Asia has title to only about one tenth of the world's wealth. Worse yet, Asia is the area of the world in which population is increasing most rapidly. The consequences are obvious.

TABLE 3

PERCENT OF WORLD's	NORTH AMERICA	ASIA
Land Surface	16%	18%
Population (1950)	9%	55%
Income (1950)	43%	12%

The per cent population increase to which I am referring throughout this talk is nothing but the difference between the death rate and the birth rate. The reason the population has increased so rapidly in many parts of the world is that rather effective death control has been practiced since the last world war, while birth control has not. In Indonesia improved death control measures have been introduced relatively recently.   Their birth rate is tremendous (in the area of 48 births per 1000 inhabitants), but their death rate is still quite high—it is two and a half or three times that of the United States. Once Indonesia's death rate decreases rapidly then its population explosion may be insurmountable.

To top this pessimistic recital, I would like to quote a very dismal sentence,[1] which will put into pespective what I want to talk about. "It is a macabre thought but a statistically accurate fact that, if an atomic bomb had been dropped on a city the size of Hiroshima every day, year in, year out, since that city was destroyed on the 6th of August, 1945, the growth in the world's population would not have been halted and in recent years would only be halved."

This is really why I want to talk about birth control. Birth control is by no means the only answer; indeed the question has been raised whether any effect can be produced fast enough with new or existing birth control procedures.   I can give you a very interesting and little known example,[2] namely Romania, which in common with many Eastern European countries has a very low birth rate. There are many reasons for it, but from an operational standpoint, the low rate was primarily maintained through legal and readily available abortion. In the year 1966 the birth rate in Romania was 13.4 per thousand, which, if compared with a country which does not practice birth control, is dramatically low, because that would be about 50 per thousand.   The Romanian government, like other Eastern European ones, became concerned about the fact that its population did not increase very much, and virtually overnight made abortion difficult. People were caught unprepared, and within 12 to 14 months the birth rate had more than doubled. Once the population had found out that abortion was not anymore easily available, it was left with two alternatives—illegal abortion, and other birth control methods. Within one year (November, 1968), the birth rate had dropped again to less than 20 per thousand.

Romania is really as dramatic an example as you can find of the impact of birth control procedures when you have a motivated population. This key point has always been made: there isn't much purpose in working on new and better birth control agents, because a population will not utilize them until it is economically motivated. The people must reach a certain level of economic development before birth control is actually used. That certainly happens to be true if one uses existing

---

[1]M. Potts, *Biologist*, 17:143, 1970.

[2]See C. Djerassi, Science and Public Affairs, Bull. Atomic Scientists 28 (No. 1), 9 (1972).

examples. For instance, among Latin American countries, Argentina is an economically highly developed country compared to Paraguay or Bolivia. In Argentina, the birth rate has been controlled through the use of existing conventional birth control agents—condoms, diaphragms, illegal abortion, etc. In contrast, its economically less well-developed neighbors have not controlled their birth rates by such procedures.

The concept that effective birth control and economic development *must* go hand in hand is a generalization that I would not necessarily buy. It certainly has applied so far to existing birth control agents, but I am not referring to existing ones. I am suggesting that whatever we need to do has to involve new agents.

In the use of new birth control agents there is one key factor that must be emphasized. It has been responsible for the spectacular and unexpectedly rapid acceptance of the only two new birth control devices that have been introduced in the last 40 years. These are the steroid oral contraceptives, which were only introduced ten years ago, and the interuterine devices, which are of even more recent origin in terms of wide use. There is one factor that is unusual about them as compared to all other birth control agents (except for abortion): contraception is separated from sexual intercourse. In my opinion, this is an indispensable prerequisite if one wants to introduce family planning and birth control quickly on a massive scale with a minimum amount of motivation. Hopefully, it could even be done in countries with a relatively low level of economic development. The reason that this has never happened before in the absence of major economic advances is that no simple contraceptive measures were available that separated birth control from sex.

CONTRACEPTION

I am the first one to agree that existing methods are not ideal. Birth control pills are not ideal because, among other things, a pill has to be taken every day. Intrauterine devices are not ideal—a certain percentage of them are expelled spontaneously, and they have a number of side effects, as do the oral contraceptives. But, so far, no one has come up with any other agents that will separate birth control from the sexual act. A year and a half ago the World Health Organization produced an excellent report[3] which summarized every theoretically feasible approach to birth control in males and females, and indicated even some of the scientific leads that were available. One conclusion that

---

[3]World Health Organization, Tech. Rep. Ser. No. 424, 1969.

can be reached from this report is that the research required is of the most sophisticated and complicated type, especially with respect to scientific manpower and finances.

The first point I would like to make, and one which I have made now in a number of talks and articles, is that we are faced with an unusual dilemma. In terms of resources, both financial and manpower, only the most technologically developed countries are in a position to carry out such research. For that reason, advances in birth control must come from areas such as North America and western Europe. Japan and the Soviet Union are technologically also equipped to create such advances, but it is interesting that, insofar as human reproductive physiology is concerned, contributions from eastern Europe have been negligible; even those from Japan have not been commensurate with her scientific potential. This may have something to do with the government policies and approaches to birth control. These are the two major areas of the world where birth control is, to a large extent, being effected through abortion, rather than exclusively through a mechanical or chemical device. These are also the only areas of the world where the use of oral contraceptive pills is not officially sanctioned.

We are thus reduced to the fact that most of the advances have come, and are bound to come in the next 10 to 20 years, from countries which are technically the most highly developed ones. Ironically, these countries (United States and western Europe) are also the ones that can most readily dispense with new birth control agents. Although we do practice birth control to a certain extent, we clearly do not do it very effectively nor to a sufficient extent. We do have a lower birth rate than many other countries. We can afford, not in the ecological sense, but at least in the sense of economic survival, a growth rate resulting in a doubling of the population every 70 years. An under-developed country, with a per capita income of $100 or $200 per year, cannot. And yet, America and some western European countries are creating more and more complicated, and even unrealistic, standards for the development of new contraceptive agents.

In part, the creation of these standards is based upon the feeling that we must not take any risks with new birth control agents, because the existing ones—condom, diaphragm, and so on—will do. I believe that this is an untenable position, because we cannot expect to develop new birth control agents and test them on the third world. It puts us in a politically and morally untenable position. This has been proven over and over again; in fact, it has been proven even in this country where the free distribution of the present birth control agents through poverty programs in the black and Puerto Rican communities is frequently asso-ciated by the inhabitants of the urban ghettos with genocidal motives.

Consequently it should not surprise us if huge populations in Asia and Africa ascribe the same motives to the European and North American governments, who preach the family planning gospel in terms of political motivation and financial support and are suggesting that the less well-developed countries use agents that we ourselves would prefer not to use. This is a ridiculous posture. The obvious response by those governments can only be averted if we are prepared to use such new agents ourselves.

As a further problem, we must realize that whatever standards we establish in the USA automatically become world standards. What we really have not done in this country, nor in western Europe, is to consider—and this is an overworked phrase now—the risk-benefit relationship between contraception and no contraception, or between good contraception and poor contraception. One can put such a risk-benefit evaluation into black and white terms. In considering the number of deaths caused by the use or lack of use of contraceptives the most serious side effect is obviously death. An equally serious side effect is the production of an unwanted child. This is really a side effect (even though it cannot be put into numerical terms) which frequently lasts with the parents for the lifetime of that child and which can have traumatic effects on the child and the parents.

In Table 4, are listed the deaths per million of women per year associated with either pregnancy or birth control procedures. If no contraceptives are used, obviously no deaths will be associated with a contraceptive agent, but one will encounter as a result of pregnancy approximately 200 to 1,000 deaths per million births. If the rhythm method is practiced, the number of deaths will be reduced to something

TABLE 4
Death rates per million women per year.
J. Goldzieher, Contraception, 1:423, 1970.

Agent	Number of Pregnancies	Total Deaths	Pregnancy Itself	Contraceptive
No Contraceptive:	800,000	200-1000	200-1000	
Rhythm Method:	230,000	60-300	60-300	None
Diaphragm:	200,000	56-280	56-280	None
Condom:	100,000	28-130	28-130	None
Intrauterine Device:	25,000	26-50	6-30	20
Oral Contraceptive:	10,000	15-40	3-15	12-24
Smoking		400		
Driving		370		

like 60 to 300 per million. With the use of a diaphragm, the number of deaths associated with pregnancy are reduced to about 56 to 280; no deaths are associated with the use of the diaphragm itself, but only with its failure as a contraceptive. If you go to a condom, which is even more effective, you find a death rate of 28 to 130—these of course are not deaths in the male, but in the female. These are again failures in terms of contraceptive efficiency, associated with pregnancy. Now, as we get to intrauterine devices, the situation starts to change. These devices are even more effective than any of the agents I have talked about so far. The number of deaths due to pregnancy is only about 20 to 50 per million. But there are a few deaths, approximately 20 in a million women, associated with the contraceptive agent itself. These result from perforation of the uterus, resulting infections, etc. Finally, there is little doubt that there are documented cases of death (12 to 20 per million) associated with the use of the oral contraceptives, primarily due to thromboembolism.

Note now that nearly 400 women per million—women of the same age group—die each year as a result of driving or smoking. Yet we are not prepared to establish standards for smoking that some would like to establish for birth control. All of you have heard, in press headlines in particular, about the tremendous number of actual (and in some cases imaginary) side effects that are associated with the use of the birth control pills. Suppose you were a new user and you were confronted with the following statement: "The pills that you will be taking are indeed more effective than any other method in preventing unwanted pregnancies, but some people may actually suffer from nausea and others occasionally from anemia and vomiting, and a few are subjected to mental confusion and some to diarrhea and occasional intestinal bleeding," and so on. If you heard a list like this, your obvious conclusion would be that one would be foolhardy to take such a pill. I think some of you may already have realized what I have done. I have not really given you some of the side effects of oral contraceptives. Rather the list of side effects is that of aspirin. In fact, if someone were to tell you that this is what aspirin does, it is unlikely that many persons would take aspirin. But this is really not how we prescribe the use of aspirin. Even the fact that aspirin is highly teratogenic[4] in rats has not stopped pregnant women from using the drug during the last 60 or 70 years, since there is no evidence that it is teratogenic in humans.

---

[4]Teratogenesis is the property of producing grossly malformed offspring; the "thalidomide babies" are a good example.

We are, however, using a completely different approach in the context of birth control agents than we do for aspirin. Incidentally, the number of deaths each year due to aspirin poisoning is on the order of 200—a small number compared to the number of people who take this drug. The same argument applies to birth control agents.

Knowing this, we now ought to turn to the question of future birth control procedures. We clearly need some new ones. Ten years ago I was extremely optimistic about the prognosis for new birth control agents. When people asked me what would happen if a woman took birth control pills for twenty years, I replied in essence, "I have no idea; it will take twenty years to determine this. But there will be no women taking them for twenty years because there will be many new and different birth control agents long before then." I am not so sure about this now. The climate with respect to research in human reproductive physiology has deteriorated tremendously during the last few years. This has happened for reasons which will become apparent in a moment.

Let us consider three different agents, at least two of which have a scientific and statistical chance of being developed. Let us start with one for the female, one on which our laboratory happens to be working quite hard. That is to develop a once-a-month pill. Clearly this is simpler than taking a pill every day. A once-a-month pill should have two effects. It should either be an abortifacient, meaning that if a woman got pregnant during the month in which she took the pill, she would simply have a chemical abortion of an embryo that would only be a few days or a few weeks old. If she were not pregnant, it should be a menses-inducing agent; that is, it would simply produce menstrual flow. Such an abortifacient or a menses-inducer would be taken approximately once a month. If we produced an ideal agent it might be active over, let's say, a period of a couple of months and a woman might have to take such a pill only if she missed a menstrual period. In other words, she may be taking only half a dozen pills per year. There are a number of obvious advantages to this, not the least of which is that the woman would not be exposed to continual therapy as she is with the present contraceptive pills.

A second contraceptive development would be a male contraceptive pill, and we shall address ourselves to the question whether a possible, scientifically feasible, approach exists.

Finally, it is conceivable that neither male nor female agent would work, perhaps because people would not be willing to take them. If the population increased at an astronomic rate, as many doomsday prophets have indicated, then you may have to have an Orwellian agent—an additive provided to food and water under government edict. These are the three chemical approaches that I would like to consider for the balance of this discussion.

These days it is easy to hear a fair number of talks, or read papers, about all the marvelous birth control agents that are just around the corner. For example, there were the well-publicized Nelson hearings in the Senate in early 1970. A question asked by one of the senators of one of the distinguished academic physicians testifying was how long would it take to develop a male contraceptive, and the reply was that we shall have one in "several years." I think this is nonsense, because most people—legislators and scientists—just have not looked seriously at the problem of what it would take to develop an agent that can be given to millions of people. It is one thing to develop one in a laboratory, but quite a different proposition to consider really putting one on the market. Therefore, I decided to determine what the requirements would be, in terms of time, money, and effort, to develop such an agent.

If you accept my premise that such agents are likely to be created only in the most highly developed countries, then you have to know what the rules of the game are in the United States, as established by the Food and Drug Administration. These happen also to be essentially the rules of the game in Western Europe. In the U. S. there are very special rules for research about birth control agents, which do not apply to any other drug. The reason for this is understandable: the FDA feels that they are dealing not with a sick population, but with a healthy one. Furthermore, the FDA is unwilling to consider some of the risks that are involved in failing to utilize birth control in the underdeveloped countries, because legally this agency is only concerned with our American milieu. And yet, as I have pointed out to you, if new agents are not developed here, they are unlikely to be developed elsewhere.

In Table 5 are summarized the special requirements which were instituted three years ago. They are quite recent, and this is why I think that the prognosis for new agents has become much poorer in recent years. On the right side of Table 5 are listed the animal requirements for the type of clinical work indicated on the left side. It should be recalled that, before any human experiments can be carried out, the physician must have approval by the Food and Drug Administration. What is called Clinical Phase I means treating only a few persons for a few days in order simply to establish what the effect is in the human. It is obvious that you first have to do some biological work in animals. The FDA requires that there be carried out three-month studies in three species of animals—rats, dogs, and monkeys. In testing other drugs, the FDA does not specify the species.

TABLE 5
Animal toxicity studies for contraceptive estrogens and progestogens.

Clinical Study	*Animal Toxicity Study Requirements*
IND PHASE I (Limited to a few subjects for up to 10 days administration)	90-Day studies in rats, dogs, and monkeys
IND PHASE II (Approximately 50 subjects for 3 menstrual cycles)	1-year studies in rats, dogs, and monkeys
IND PHASE III (Clinical Trial)	2-year studies in rats, dogs, and monkeys. Initiation of 7-year dog and 10-year monkey studies prior to start of Phase 3. Reproduction and teratology studies in 2 species.
NDA (New Drug Application)	No further requirements, but must include up-to-date progress on long-term dog and monkey studies.

Phase II clinical work means actually testing the agent in about 50 people, in order to determine whether it is really effective, and to determine the dose. Before you are permitted to do this for contraceptive agents, you must have completed one-year studies in, again, rats, dogs, and monkeys. Before you can do real clinical work to determine the efficacy, you must have completed two-year studies in, again, these three species, and you must have underway ten-year studies in monkeys and seven-year studies in dogs. These requirements are quite unprecedented in magnitude; however, the rationale seems reasonable if you want to protect the public. But are you really protecting the public? The only reason why one carries out animal experiments is, of course, to save research time and to reduce the possibility of damage to humans. Therefore, one should select an animal that is relevant to the human. Both the rat, and particularly the dog, are essentially irrelevant examples as far as human reproduction is concerned. The use of specified animals is the most serious objection—it is one which has not been publicized enough. In order to carry out research on contraceptives, you have to do it in these three particular animals, and particularly the dog. Use of the dog has been responsible for some very tragic reversals in recent years. There have now been five contraceptive agents that have already been stopped in clinical investigation, or withdrawn from the market, as a result of experiments on dogs, even though they were devoid of similar side effects in humans. The reasons that the dog is a poor example are several. First, such animal experiments are carried out as models for contraceptive trials in women. The woman goes through a menstrual cycle roughly every month. The bitch goes into heat only twice a year. The monkey, incidentally (particularly the higher ape), has a menstrual cycle similar to that of the human. Secondly, dogs are notoriously sensitive to steroids, much more so than monkeys and human beings.

We really ought to pick as models species that are more closely related to humans. Table 6 presents some interesting experiments that have been carried out recently on a new drug in order to see what the best animal model would be for eventual clinical trial. This happens to be a drug which, in man, is secreted largely in the urine, hardly at all in the feces and whose plasma half-life is approximately 14 hours. Below this entry in Table 6 are listed seven different animal species including the rat, the guinea pig, and the dog; three species of monkeys; and a new species which has been used recently in toxicology, the mini-pig, which is not a guinea pig but rather a pig with the approximate weight and body surface of an adult human.

TABLE 6
Excretion patterns and plasma half-life of an experimental drug.

Species	Excretion Urine %	Excretion Feces %	Plasma Half Life Hours
Man	94	1 - 2	14
Rat	90	2	4 - 6
Guinea Pig	90	5	9
Dog	29	50	23 - 35
Rhesus Monkey[1]	90	2	2 - 3
Capuchin Monkey	45	54	20
Stump Tail Monkey[1]	40	60	1
Mini-Pig	86	1 - 2	4 - 7

[1] These two species belong to the same genus *(Macaca)*.

Now look at what animal actually resembles man most closely in this case. If you examine urinary excretion, then the mini-pig and the rat are much closer to man, for instance, than the dog. Even more interesting are the three species of monkeys. This is very important, because people just assume that a monkey is a monkey, and that is simply not true. The Rhesus monkey, in terms of excretion, resembles a human. The Capuchin monkey, or the Stumptail monkey, which incidentally is very similar to the Rhesus monkey in other respects, is very different metabolically. Even more important is the question of plasma half-life. It turns out that the mini-pig is probably the best animal model in this case, all things being taken equally. It is perfectly obvious, therefore, that if you want to pick an animal model you have to pick one that is suitable for the particular drug and which resembles man closely. It would be absurd to follow some bureaucratic rule which requires, for instance, that one must select a rat and a dog, for instance, rather than the mini-pig and the monkey.

It would be even better if we could use higher apes which, of course, are closer to human beings. Here you encounter complications with respect to cost. A Rhesus monkey costs about $100. Even the small apes, such as the baboon, cost about $200. The price of a chimpanzee is $1,000, and a gorilla costs anywhere from $2,000 to $5,000. You can imagine what the additional costs are in terms of housing and handling. Furthermore, the number of animals that are required is enormous. Since we do not know how to breed apes, we would be likely to exterminate them very quickly if we collected them at the rate at which we are, for instance, now collecting Rhesus monkeys. This is one of the biggest bottlenecks in reproductive biology research: we do not have enough primates and primate colonies. We really do not have enough information or enough good animal models to create new contraceptive procedures that are applicable to human beings. This is one of our most serious problems. It is one which neither the FDA, nor the public, nor, for that matter, even many scientists, have considered sufficiently.

The second point to consider is that the FDA is the protector of the consumer. I think it should be so. It is very important that an independent government agency looks out for the consumer, insofar as agents are concerned that are or will be on the market. But since 1962 the FDA has acquired a second legal function; it is, in essence, also the controller of clinical research in this country. In other words, it has become both a policeman, on the one hand, and a stimulator, if you wish, of research, on the other hand. I think these are two conflicting roles which are very difficult to fulfill. The FDA has done some very unwise things in terms of scientific decisions. I gave you one example—this sudden requirement that the dog has to be used as a model for humans in contraceptives. There is no appeal procedure to such scientific decisions of the FDA. One of my first proposals therefore would be that there should be some independent scientific body, such as the National Academy of Sciences or the World Health Organization, to which one could appeal for research decisions which have nothing to do with the consumer. This is important, for these rules do not pertain to agents that are put on the market; they pertain to agents that are about to be subjected to clinical research scrutiny.

The next question that we should consider is how much it will cost to develop such an agent, and, before we do so, from where the money will come. Apparently very little has been done about determining how much money has been spent on contraceptive research. The government had spent practically nothing on research for new birth control agents prior to the early 1960's. Most research in this field during the 1950's was supported by only three pharmaceutical companies. It was only when the first oral contraceptive pills were put on the market around 1960, and when the urgency of the population problem was well publicized, that government funds started to become available. In the years 1969 and 1970 the NIH, through a special center for contraceptive research, allocated 12.5 million dollars, of which 9 million dollars will be used for contraceptive research. The Ford Foundation has probably spent more than any other nonindustrial group—something on the order of $7 to 10 million per year; industry—no one knew.

Therefore I decided to contact five different pharamceutical companies that have been active in this field, and ask them if they could tell me how much money they have spent for birth control research in the last five years. It turned out that these five U. S. companies alone had spent $68 million in these five years. There were several American and European companies that I had not asked, so that a conservative figure for industry expenditures is probably $100 million in the last five years, which is more than has been spent anywhere else by any public or nonprofit agency. In a way this is very unfortunate, because, in my opinion, it is really very important that much more money come from the public sector. The point I want to make is that so far it has not come from there and, what is even more important, the incentive for industry to spend such amounts in the future is becoming less all the time.

What does it take to develop a new, once-a-month pill for the female? In Figure 2 I have constructed a critical path map (CPM) for such a birth control agent. I have done this in the context of what is required, not only by government, but also by scientific requirements. The start of our project is number 1, and our final aim is the point number 9, at which an agent can be distributed to the public. The figures below each line are the number of months—and these are very optimistic estimates. I have drawn here a chart which is an idealized one, since it assumed perfect coordination and perfect telescoping whenever possible.

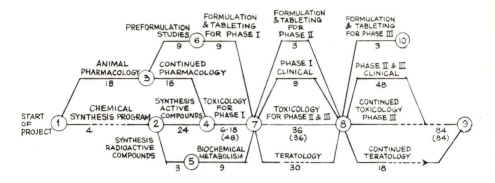

Figure 2: Basic critical path map for a luteolytic or abortifacient agent. Total time (including NDA file preparation) 126 to 210 months. Cost: $7 - $18 million.

The first step is the chemical synthesis of a new compound. While compounds are being synthesized, one already starts animal experiments, within the same period of time. The most promising candidates from such pharmacological screening are already subjected to two further procedures. First, synthesis of radioactive analogs because we must know something about the metabolic handling of the compound in order to carry out studies (Table 6) to find out which animal is the proper model, and whether it resembles the human. At the same time you have to start some formulation studies in order to even know how to give it to the human being—you do not just put it in a pill. If you coordinate all of these things in the manner which I have shown in Figure 1 and, in the meanwhile, continue pharmacology, you can, for the most promising compounds, start the initial toxicology. In a number of cases, the toxicology needs to take at least one year. While you do such toxicology you can, if you wish, start preparations for the Phase I clinical trial. If you are willing to gamble, you continue the longer toxicology. In the meanwhile you start something which I have put down here as teratology. Teratology is to indicate what happens to the embryo if, in fact, there is a failure in the method. This is of crucial importance. If you use an abortifacient, or a pill that a woman takes once a month, it may fail. There will be a few cases where it is bound to fail. The question that you will ask, obviously, is what will happen if the child is born. Will it be a malformed child or will it be a normal one? Even if this method fails in only 0.1 per cent it could mean that one child out of every thousand could be a thalidomide-type child. You know perfectly well that this would be totally unacceptable. You have to determine this, and about the only reasonable animal for human experiments would be the monkey. Teratology could be done in humans directly, if you wish, by aborting surgically all failures. In fact, you will probably have to do this.

Suppose you finally have an agent which is a candidate for extensive human trial. In order to determine the effective dose you will have to continue to lower the amount given until you reach a dose at which you have some failures. If you have failures, what do you do? The best thing, in fact, is to abort them surgically. If you want to get the maximum amount of information, you would be wise not to abort them until past the twelfth to fourteenth week, because by that time the fetus will be sufficiently developed that when you abort it you can actually determine whether there has been any malformation. The number of women who would be willing to subject themselves to this type of experiment is relatively limited, because an abortion during the second trimester is much more serious than a simple abortion in the early stages of pregnancy. The number of states in which you could carry out such experiments in the United States is extremely limited. In fact, just a couple of years ago, it would have been impossible to carry out such experimentation in the United States. This is one of the complications that I indicated in the beginning. Where will you carry out such experiments, if you do not carry them out here?

You need to do these things before you get into Phase II and Phase III clinical work. If you add up all the months that I have given to you, and if you superimpose on these the FDA requirements of long term animal toxicology which I summarized in Table 5, you come up with a total of 126 to 210 months.

Now 126 months is over ten years, which places us already at 1980. That would mean that if you want to have an agent in 1980, it would have to exist in the laboratory right now. Moreover, it would have to be in the laboratory of an absolutely ideal organization, which most certainly is not a university, or a hospital, or even a government laboratory. Where will you be able to carry out this coordination I have just indicated? This is where the role of the pharmaceutical industry comes in.

To my knowledge, no drug has been developed, since 1940, by a hospital, a medical school, or a government agency, either in Western Europe, the United States, or Japan. This doesn't mean that some of the work has not been done in a medical school or by scientists in universities. It does mean that in order to put all these things together, and really to coordinate them, a type of entrepreneurial and organizational talent is required which so far is seen only in industry.

There is one alternative, and that is to socialize the process. This has been done in Eastern Europe. For the purposes of our discussion, it does not matter whether such an agent is produced by socialized industry or through private enterprise. The only point that I want to make is that one or the other will have to do it. If we are prepared to do it through a socialized route, then I think that we should take the steps that are necessary to organize such a system. That would mean, incidentally, that the cost figures that I talked about here would probably have to be doubled or tripled. The cost figure that I have calculated in Figure 2, which is on the order of $7 to $18 million for one such agent, presupposes that you already have all the organization set up. If you have to set it up, the drug obviously will have to cost very much more, maybe between five and ten times the cost figure for an already running system. That is still not an enormous figure by comparison to the SST, for instance, but it is an unprecedented figure for the development of any drug.

In Figures 3 and 4, I have shown the steroids which correspond to the chemical structures of the presently used oral contraceptive pills.

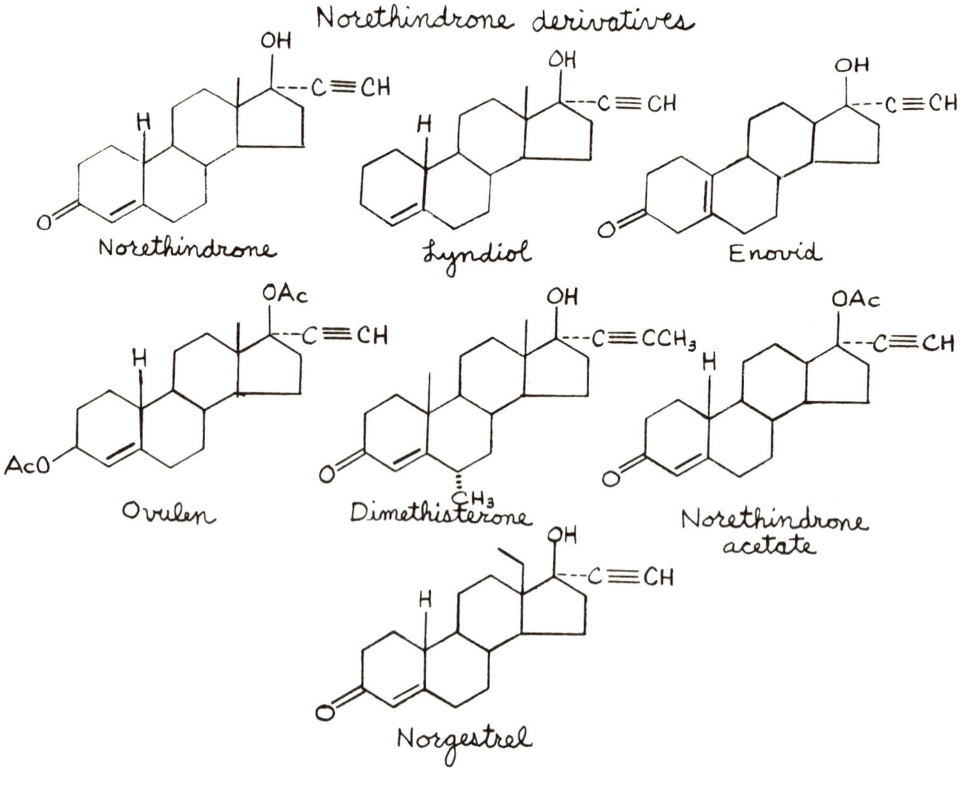

Figure 3: Norethindrone derivatives.

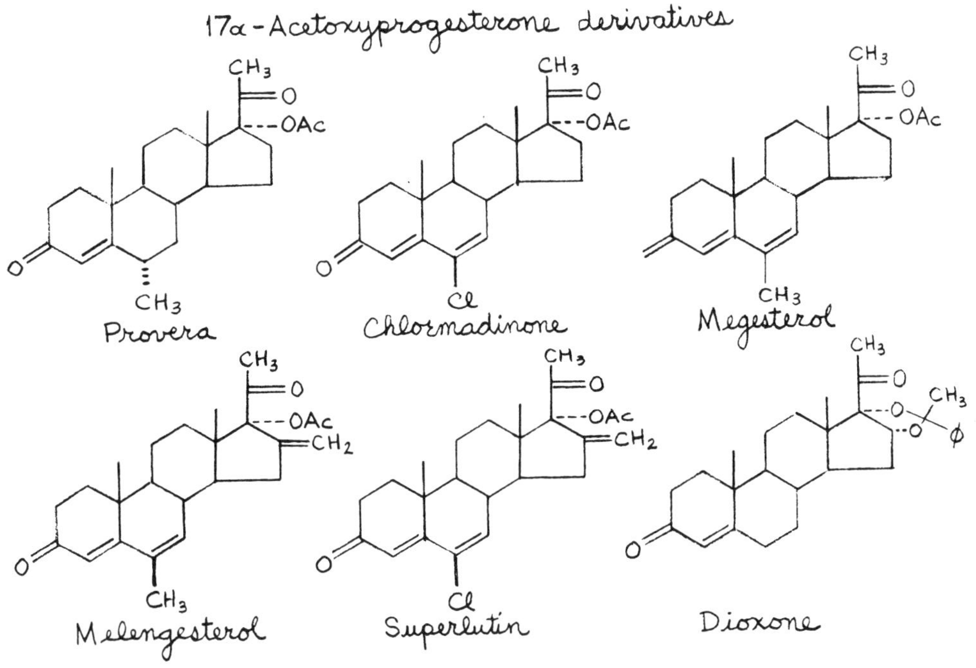

Figure 4: *17a-Acetoxyprogesterone derivatives.*

If you are a steroid chemist you will appreciate the subtleties. If you are not one then they will probably all look more or less the same to you. You may have read recently about a new development with prostaglandins. The structures of three of them are shown in Figure 5. You will notice that they are completely different from steroids—chemically rather simpler. The newspapers have indicated that these are a great breakthrough in contraceptive technology. I think they represent a

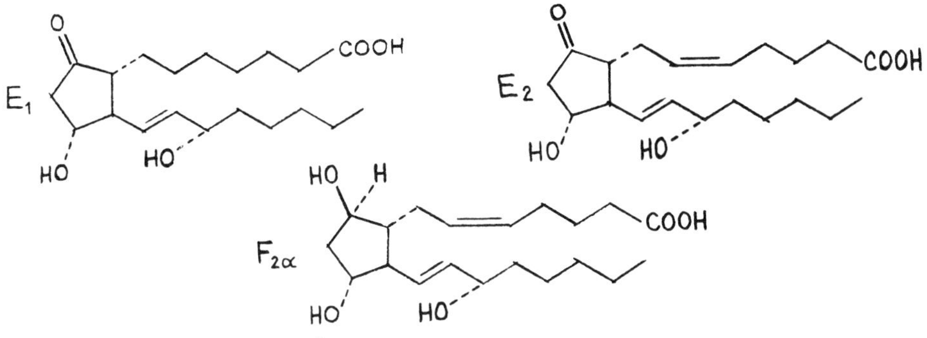

Figure 5: *Three prostaglandins.*

potential one, but I doubt whether the public realizes what the time requirements are before they become every-day drugs.

Table 7 is taken from a meeting of the New York Academy of Sciences in September, 1970, and describes work done by a group in Sweden, where much of the research on prostaglandins has been pioneered. These happen to be very interesting compounds which actually do produce abortion. This is really a chemical abortifacient, although

TABLE 7
Use of phostaglandin F_{2a} for abortion

Week of Gestation	No. of Subjects Failures.	Infusion Time (Hrs.)	Total Dose (mg)	No. of Completed Abortions
< 8	22/2	7.6	31.1	20
9 - 12	19/13	13.4	61.8	6
13 - 15	18/16	13.2	70.9	2
> 16	10/8	13.9	66.7	2

its biological mechanism is quite different from what another abortifacient might do. Notice the number of subject failures: in 22 patients there were only 2 failures when they took women that were eight weeks or less pregnant. But as they went up to more than 16 weeks of pregnancy, 8 out of 10 were failures. More recent work has shown that, using different routes of administration and dose regimens, the success rate in second trimester abortions may reach 50 per cent. In other words, this is a potentially good agent at the early stages of pregnancy, but not a very good one at late stages. But the problems are, we do not yet know what happened during the failures, and a great deal of teratology needs to be done.

Even more serious is the fact that so far the prostaglandins have only been active by infusion over 12 to 70 hours, and not orally. You can well appreciate that to have an abortifacient which women can use, particularly in underdeveloped countries, it would have to be active either by mouth, or, possibly, by insertion into the uterus or vagina, but quite clearly not by long-term infusion. In order to create an orally effective abortifacient—no one has done so yet—one is literally at the beginning of the CPM chart of Figure 3. I just want to point out that before prostaglandins are going to be orally or generally used abortifacients, one is really quite far behind.

Let us now consider the proposal for male contraceptives. The statement has frequently been made, only partly tongue in cheek, that the reason why all of the recently developed contraceptive devices are applicable to the female is that virtually all of the research is being done by men. Actually, it turns out that we know very much more about the female reproductive system than we know about the male reproductive system and, at this time, it is easier to develop a contraceptive agent for the female than the male. There are many more places in which you can interfere with the female reproductive system: ovulation, mobility of the egg, implantation, embryogenesis, and, of course, abortion. This is by no means the case with the male. We know much less about the male reproductive system. A second reason which has been often overlooked is the difficulty in clinical work. Consider for a moment how you would do research on men. How do you do it in women, incidentally? It is relatively simple. When a woman is pregnant, and she does not want to remain pregnant, she has a real motivation to do something about it. She really has physical consequences to bear, in addition to the possible economic ones. I am mentioning also the economic ones because again taking Latin America as an example, well over 50 per cent of the children born in these countries are illegitimate children for whom the man carries no responsibility. You can reach women through Planned Parenthood Associations, and you can reach them through gynecologists and obstretricians. This is not where you can get men. In fact, if a man in our society goes anywhere with sexual problems or reproductive problems, he goes primarily to a psychiatrist. That is really not the place where you go to find experimental models for reproduction. This is one of the really serious problems in research on contraceptives in males—their preoccupation with potency and sexual performance, and the fear that almost any agent that affects their reproductive organs will, in fact, interfere with sexual potency. I am convinced that, if we are going to produce a practical male contraceptive pill, we will have to show that it also increases libido.

Where do we find male volunteers for such purposes? You can find them in only two places: a prison or the army. There is one common factor about these situations—you do not have any women around. Therefore you are reduced, to a large extent, to examining masturbation samples of sperm. That is already a more indirect experiment, and clearly not one which really tests the eventual applicability and acceptability. Eventually one must determine what happens in actual concrete trials. This is certainly what happens in female contraceptive testing. When women are exposed to contraceptives one eventually determines what happens to the birth rate—to the number of pregnancies. This is the proof of the pudding. Furthermore, it turns out that in the entire United States there happen to be no more than two to three clinical centers that would be equipped to carry out clinical research on male contraceptives, compared to literally dozens of clinical centers where reproductive clinical research on females can be carried out. That is a tremendous difficulty.

Finally, there is a great difficulty about the receptivity of the male for using such agents. If I were a woman I would not really want to depend on the male having taken the pill unless we are dealing with monogamous relationships of fairly highly motivated people. If one is talking about birth control in an occasional sexual relationship, where the woman may be in contact with a particular man and not see him again, where he will literally not care what happens to her, then it is absolutely crucial that she know that he actually put the pill in his mouth and swallowed it.

However, there is one important advantage to a male contraceptive that should not be underestimated. If you had a male contraceptive similar to the female one, it would have to be taken, let's say, every day. In a monogamous, or in a permanent or semipermanent relationship, the man and the woman could alternate. The woman could take her pill for three to six months, and then she could stop, and the man could take his for such a period of time. That would be an important extra because it would eliminate the most important drawback of the present oral contraceptives in females—their continued, long-term use.

How long will it take to develop a male contraceptive? Figure 6 shows the critical path map for a male contraceptive pill. I only want to point out to you that, because you have many fewer leads and the clinical work takes longer, the minimum time is probably 150 months, and a closer estimate is somewhere around 200 to 240 months. This is,

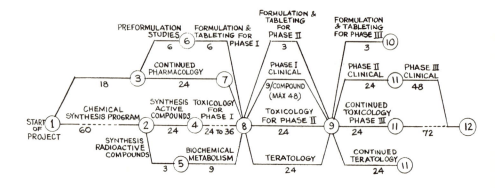

Figure 6: Critical path map for development of a male antifertility agent. Total time (including NDA file preparation) 150-246 months. Cost: $6-? million.

of course, where the 1984 in my title enters again. There is hardly a chance of having such an agent before the 1980's. If you are fantastically lucky and everything goes right, and you do not have to do the type of long-term toxicology that I outlined in Table 5, it might be accomplished for $6 million. I think this is unlikely, and a closer figure would probably be something on the order of $30 million. The questions are: Who will put out the money, and where will it be done?

Let me go now to the last type of agent, namely, the Orwellian additive to food and water. There have been statements made in the literature that within five to fifteen years we will have such an agent. Let's consider for a moment, not what it takes or what it costs, but what such an agent actually ought to do. You have two choices. You can add it to food or you can add it to water. Let's consider food; since this is going to be an agent added by government edict, the supplier of the food will have to put it in, not the consumer. What foodstuff would you use? You can't use things like peanut butter, because you will find people like myself who hate peanut butter with a passion. There is really only one foodstuff that, in essense, you cannot do without, and that happens to be salt. So one possibility would be to add it to salt. But suppose we do that. We're not going to have salt for men and salt for women and salt for children or old people. Therefore, we shall have to develop an agent that will be tolerated by males and females, by old people, and by young people, but that will be effective in only one sex. Let's say it will be a male contraceptive, so it will be active only on males. It really ought to be active on males only during the reproductive years—it should not effect the male reproductive organs during puberty or adolescence. It will have to be effective over an enormous dose range, because you will have a 20 pound child taking it, and you may have a 250 pound man taking it. You have someone who eats a lot at one meal, very little at another one. Some people like to put a lot of salt on food, others use very little. This is almost an inconceivable dose requirement for an agent. In addition, it is not supposed to have any side effects, since we are not even prepared to tolerate the side effects of the present oral contraceptive, and these are pretty minimal by comparison to what I am talking about here.

The drug will have to be tasteless, it should resist boiling, it should resist freezing, food preservation, enormous temperature ranges, and it should be stable over long periods of time. I could go on, but it is pretty obvious that something along these lines will not be developed during the next 15 years or even in this century.

Let's say we put it into water. There is one problem right away, and that is that at least half the world's population, and maybe even more than that, do not drink their water from a central water supply.

They take it out of wells or rivers, about which you can do nothing. Suppose we even forget about these and use it only for that population that takes water from central supplies. We again have to fulfill all these requirements; it has to be tasteless, water soluble, resistant to boiling, freezing, it shouldn't precipitate out during food concentration, and so on. In addition, if you have such an agent, you are not talking anymore about a contaminant of the person's microecology, you are talking about a general pesticide. In this case we are talking about a pesticide against humans, but it is one that really will be applied to animals also, because they drink the same water. You won't want to exterminate an animal population, so you have to find an additive which is specific to humans and not to animals. Notice that this is, by definition, impossible, if you carry out your first experiments on animal subjects. Unless you decide to do your screening first in humans, and then, when you find an agent that is active in humans, apply it to animals, it is just impossible to come up with such an agent. Suppose even that all these things happen—then you have to find a second agent that people will buy, or get on license, which will reverse these effects. And that agent will have to have practically the same properties. Well, that is just impossible—certainly in this century, certainly with the limitations of time and manpower and everything else that I have mentioned.

My conclusion is a fairly dismal one. We are boxing ourselves into a corner. We are establishing conditions for research in the contraceptive field that make it progressively more difficult and less likely that such research in humans will be carried out, and yet the need for such agents grows greater all the time. The immediate answer is that of the informed citizen in the highly developed countries. It was public pressure, promoted through a sensational press, that led to legislative pressures upon government agencies such as the FDA. These agencies have created rules and regulations that are, perhaps, realistic within the confines of the American consumer, but totally unrealistic in the world-wide context of the population problem—and yet, this is a world problem. Unless we are going to have public pressures that will, first, change or in some way alter the way in which we carry out research in this field, and, second, create financial resources of a much larger scale than we have right now available, than the prospects of developing the sort of agent that I have been talking about, even in the 1980's, are dim.

SUGGESTED READING

Berelson, B., Beyond Family Planning, Science, 163:533, 1969.

Westoff, C. F., and Bumpass, L., The Revolution in Birth Control Practices of U. S. Roman Catholics, Science, 179:41, 1973.

Hardin, G., Population, Evolution, and Birth Control, San Francisco, W. H. Freeman, 2nd Edition, 1969.

WHO CARES WHERE THEY COME DOWN

Relevance Revisited

John R. Lombardi

> " 'Once the rockets are up
> Who cares where they come down
> That's not my department,'
> Says Wernher von Braun.''[1]

Since our technological success in World War II with everything from radar to the atomic bomb, the United States has been on what must be regarded as a scientific binge. Stimulated by competition with Russia, congressional and public opinion were dazzled with the promise of global security and better living through chemistry. Exponential increases in scientific research budgets fed the enormous expansion of graduate education. Lost among the growing clamor for scientific funding were a few meek voices asking "Is science really relevant?" Although this question nagged a few scattered individuals, it was largely ignored by the scientific community. Nevertheless, an increasing chorus of individuals both within and outside science began to make the question more and more a part of the growing debate over national priorities and the quality of life in the United States. Perhaps a watershed was reached in the Spring of 1970, in the wake of the Cambodia-Kent State demonstrations, when the scientific establishment as well as the government came under severe attack. Scientists could no longer afford to ignore the question of relevancy.

As a response, several faculty members at the University of Illinois, including myself, decided to assemble a series of lectures designed to answer the question "Is Chemistry Relevant?" It is, of course, that series which has led to the present book. It is my honest

---

[1] T. Lehrer.

opinion that this series has been, overall, a dismal failure. First I would like to say that I am not criticizing the quality of the talks here transcribed to articles, nor the research described, which on the whole I consider quite good. What I am criticizing is the implied definition which has been attached to "relevance." Many of the subjects presented assume that mere solution of technological problems may be equated with relevance. I hope here to broaden this definition of relevance and to gain a clearer idea of how our responsibilities as scientists relate to the meaning of relevance.

The first thing I would like to convince you of is that scientific relevance cannot simply be equated with the solution of technological problems. Let us consider some examples.

First, the problem of defoliation in Viet Nam. We have had a recurring argument at the University of Illinois concerning the morality of working for the Department of Defense. Rather than revive that argument, I would like to concede, for the sake of argument, that it is legitimate, and could even be considered relevant, to work for the Department of Defense. Instead, consider the history of the chemical 2,4,5-T, a defoliant widely used in Viet Nam by our armed forces to remove leaves from trees, to make the enemy more visible, and to destroy crops to make the enemy more hungry.[2] By 1965 over 40 million pounds of 2,4,5-T had been sprayed over forest and cropland, destroying over 5 per cent of South Viet Nam's foliage. In late 1967 numerous Saigon newspapers carried stories about an increasingly common birth defect described as "egg-bundle-like fetus." The increases were all detected near areas recently sprayed with the defoliant. Due to this and other more scientific tests on animals, 2,4,5-T has been banned for use near populated areas and on crops for human consumption in the United States. Later, an impurity, dioxin, was found in separate tests to be highly poisonous and teratogenic. But how did it come to pass that we used a potential teratogen, which can harm a fetus much more than an enemy, so extensively in Viet Nam? Imagine a military man or politician approaching a scientist asking for a defoliant. The scientist replies "Here, I've got just the thing for you on my shelf—2,4,5-T," or perhaps he asks for laboratory equipment to find one. Did the scientist test his product for impurities? Did he examine the side effects that were possible? It could be that the military program could not wait. Did the scientist try to make the military men or politicians aware of the possibility that there were impurities or side effects? Can the military be expected to ask about these effects without some

---

[2]Another view of the problems posed by 2,4,5-T is provided in the article by Julius Johnson in this book, "To Weed or Not to Weed ".

education about chemistry? Yes, the scientist solved a technological problem; he found a defoliant, but is that alone sufficient?

As a second example, I had originally planned to discuss the effects of technology on our ecology. However, this topic has been covered very thoroughly by Barry Commoner.[3] I'll just summarize briefly how his remarks fit into what I have to say. One could, for example, consider working on aluminum to replace steel, synthetics such as nylon to replace cotton, or detergents to replace soap, all problems regarded as relevant. All of these things make life more comfortable and somewhat cheaper. But Dr. Commoner has noted that we pay a pretty high long-run price for a short-run gain. He warns of an impending ecological crisis in this country as a result of techno-logical developments. The reason is that we have violated an eco-logical law which, briefly stated, is "Everything has to go somewhere." Relevant science must conform to all scientific laws, not just those laws that tend to maximize profit or convenience. If we invent some-thing it must obey the laws of thermodynamics if it is going to work, and clearly it will also have to obey the laws of ecology if we are to survive.

A third example is pollution. Many of our discussions have con-cerned either statements of, or technological solutions to, the problems of air and water pollution. Much money is available now to work on this and it is considered very "relevant" work. I am not criticizing people who work on pollution, but I question its relevance in the follow-ing sense; I have absolutely no doubt that the problem will be solved—the only real question I have is, Who will pay? And the answer is that it will be the taxpayers and consumers, not the people who profit from pollution. Pollution problems will be solved by tax rebates for in-dustries, which means higher rates for the average taxpayer. The tax-payer will pay through government sponsored research, and, of course, industry-sponsored research will be passed along to the taxpayer and consumer through higher prices, keeping profits at the same level. In addition, industrial research will be tax deductible. We must recognize that the profit system encourages pollution, but it is not going to eliminate pollution; the taxpayers are.

I am sure you can think of many more examples, but it is clear to me that these examples suffice to disprove any necessary connection between the solution of technological problems and relevance. In all three cases—defoliation, ecology, and pollution—technological solutions alone were not enough. We all know the old maxim that every solution to a problem creates more problems. I would like to put forth the thesis

---

[3]See "The Environmental Cost of Economic Growth" by Barry Commoner.

that *every technological solution creates a human problem.* I am sure
we will discover this to be true if we examine history, going back to
the discovery of fire, through the printing press, right up to atomic
energy. One might reply that it is not a scientist's job to make a value
judgment. His only job is to make accurate scientific measurements,
and all his responsibilities stop there. The song composed and recorded by Tom Lehrer, an excerpt from which begins this article, records
what one graduate student thought of this attitude.

The song is partly in fun, but nevertheless I find that the attitude
"It's not my department" is extremely prevalent among scientists.
Somehow they feel that the human problems created by their technological solutions should be dealt with by someone else; that scientists
do not make value judgments. I maintain that this is not true. Consider, for example, a very eminent and brilliant organic chemist, Louis
Fieser. He has to his credit many great scientific achievements. However, one of his more notorious is the development of napalm, which
he worked on during World War II. Recently he was asked how he feels
about the use of his invention now that it is used extensively against
civilians in Viet Nam. His reply was that he feels no guilt. "That is
for other people. I was working on a technological problem that was
considered pressing." It sounds as if he is not making a value judgment. However, he considered this technological problem more pressing
than any possible misuse or side effects. That is a value judgment.

Another example of this type of thinking came out in the recent
controversy at the University of Illinois over Illiac IV. Illiac IV was a
computer, to be paid for by the Department of Defense, which would be
designed and run by scientists on this campus. The Department of
Defense would have obtained two-thirds of the user time and one-third
could have been used by University scientists for "worthy projects."
Daniel Slotnick, who was the major innovator and in charge of the
project, said, "misuses represented by the DOD role are subtracted
from advantages and it will come out plus, but to limit technology because of detrimental side effects is ridiculous." Whether you agree or
disagree with this statement, you must admit it represents a value
judgment; technology is so important that side effects may be ignored.

The scientific ideal is not to make a value judgment. However,
in practice we make them all the time. Even the act of refusing to make
a value judgment is itself a value judgment. On a day-to-day basis
when we decide whether to work on tomorrow's lecture or do some
research, it is a value judgment. When we choose to work on one
research project over another, that is a value judgment. When we
choose which aspect of a particular problem to emphasize in print or
when talking to colleagues, such as the defoliant nature of 2,4,5-T or

its side effects, we are making a value judgment. And with the increasing dependence of society on technology, the results of scientific value judgments are becoming more and more important.

One example of this is the widely-held idea that computers are somehow impartial. Many people think that if a computer is used anywhere along the line in analyzing statistics, the result must be unbiased and accurate. You have probably seen on election night, as results come in, a large computer bank behind Huntley and Brinkley. Very early, around 6 p.m., the inevitable election results are announced. The computer supposedly works this out. Actually some political scientist sat down, analyzed all previous results and put a weight or value on the results of each precinct; on the basis of these weights the computer multiplies the early returns by the proper factors and predicts the results. The results are not impartial at all, but reflect all the biases and values the programmer put in.

Another deceptive thing about computers is significant figures. A computer calculates a number to eight digits, and when someone sees so many digits it is very tempting to believe more of them than are really meaningful. Of course, the Madison Avenue advertising agencies have taken this over. One often sees advertisements which state something like "81.8 per cent of doctors polled prefer Brand A." Perhaps only 11 doctors were polled and 9 preferred Brand A, but the number 81.8 per cent implies far more significance than can really be attached to the poll.

I think it is clear to everyone that the symbiotic bond between science and society has grown tighter in the last few decades. The American public has been seduced by the possibility of technological solutions to the growing maze of problems which confront our increasingly complex society. Scientists have willingly fostered the idea that all problems can be solved given enough money and know-how. Yet as technology grows more complex, some of the requirements of society tend to clash through their separate and contradictory technological extensions. At this point, some of the technological solutions must fail, and society, believing in the ultimate capabilities of science, has not been prepared to comprehend the meaning and genesis of this breakdown. We are now experiencing just the beginning of public disillusionment with technological solutions. Part of the responsibility for this situation rests squarely on our shoulders. It was easy to sell congressmen and the press on the wondrous rewards which lay in store if research were only funded. It was much more difficult to express, in addition, the limitations, contradictions, and possible side effects of scientific advancement. It was more difficult and it was not done. Now we are paying the price.

It is time for scientists to face up to some of our other responsibilities. Could a military man or politician have the scientific knowledge to question if there were possible side effects to 2,4,5-T? Does a corporate executive understand ecology? Does the average citizen know how to dispute the findings of a computer? Are consumers conversant with all the ways advertisers can lie with statistics? Does the average citizen know the real uncertainties and ambiguities we face every day in the laboratory? Many people have an image of a scientist putting on a clean white coat every day and making precise measurements with precise instruments. Any of us who have ever conducted any research know this is a deception. It is rare that a scientist is ever 100 per cent sure of his results. There are numerous uncertainties and ambiguities, and anyone who doesn't recognize this should take a closer look at his work.

What then are our real responsibilities as scientists? Our first responsibility, of course, is to do good science, and we all know that. I think we must go farther. We must ourselves recognize, and we must communicate to the society around us, the necessary limitations which accompany technological development. We must recognize that technological solutions are not synonymous with relevance, but in fact create human problems. If this statement is accepted, it follows necessarily that scientists make value judgments. We must face this fact and thereby help the public correctly interpret the implications of technological advances. This means communicating our feelings as to possible side effects, our doubts as to the certainty of our results, and our questions and apprehensions about possible misuse of science. We must also learn about those human problems which are created by our solutions, not that we alone can solve these problems, but that we can work with society to better explain and search for truly relevant problems.

SUGGESTED READING

President's Science Advisory Board: Report on 2,4,5-T, Washington, D.C., U.S. Government Printing Office, March, 1971. (Price $0.40; write to the Superintendent of Documents.)

Einstein, A., Essays in Science, New York, The Philosophical Library, Inc., 1933.

Lundberg, F., The Rich and the Super-Rich, New York, Bantam Books, 1968.

Mills, C. W., The Power Elite, New York, Oxford University Press, 1956.

SPEAK TRUTH TO POWER

John E. Baldwin

The prospect of discussing at the University of Illinois the formal apparatus through which the President receives advice on technical issues was a little terrifying. Many other members of that academic community know much more about the topic than I do. Over the past several decades the University of Illinois has provided a large fraction of the expertise and advice in the physical sciences made available to the various departments of the executive branch of our Federal Government.

I will, however, try to describe the official channels and institutional arrangements through which the President of the United States receives technical advice. I shall also mention some closely related topics, including some apparent weaknesses in the system as it is currently structured and operated.

THE MACHINERY OF ADVICE

The first formal designation of a Science Advisor to a President came in November, 1957, one month after the epoch-making flight of Sputnik. President Eisenhower chose James R. Killian, Jr. to be his Special Assistant for Science and Technology. Killian also became chairman of a President's Science Advisory Committee. In 1962, the PSAC and the Office of Science and Technology were put in their

217

present form. Together they provide the formal institutional mechanism for generating analysis and opinion on technical issues and for communicating advice to the President through his Science Advisor.

The PSAC is composed of the Science Advisor, presently Dr. Edward E. David, Jr., and 16 others having expertise in science and engineering. They come from both academic and industrial backgrounds, and usually have both technical and administrative experience. They are appointed by the President for staggered, four-year terms. They usually meet two days each month.

Within PSAC there is concentrated a breadth of experience, perspective, and viewpoint on issues having significant scientific or technical components. PSAC is aided by the staff of the Office of Science and Technology in Washington and by its subcommittees or panels.

The Office of Science and Technology (OST) is an Executive Agency, staffed by about 70 full-time employees. Approximately one-fourth are professionals with scientific backgrounds who provide guidance to the President on technical issues on a day-to-day basis.

The National Academy of Sciences (NAS) and the National Research Council may, when asked to do so, undertake studies and formulate recommendations on specific issues. The prestige of the Academy is such that it is able to recruit relatively quickly competent specialists to serve on *ad hoc* study panels. Their recommendations are by no means always transformed into public policy, but they do carry special weight.

There are other scientific advisory groups attached to specific parts of the executive branch. The Departments of Health, Education and Welfare; Commerce; Transportation; Defense; and others seek advice appropriate to their particular responsibilities. Such advice, after being considered by the administrative and political leadership of a Department, may become a contributing element in a policy recommendation made by that Department to the White House.

The Science Advisor, in addition to his roles as personal advisor to the President, chairman of the PSAC, and Director of the Office of Science and Technology, is also chairman of the Federal Council on Science and Technology, which attempts to provide some interagency correlation of federal programs in this area.

The subcommittees of the PSAC are working groups, typically chaired by a member of PSAC and comprised of academic and industrial consultants, men having some technical capacity or subject specialty considered relevant to the problems under discussion.

The range of topics discussed at the PSAC subcommittee level may be gleaned from a partial list of published reports, or a listing of panels now in operation, Pesticides (1963); Restoring the Quality of the Environment (1965), Toxicological Information and Drug Safety (1966), Post-Apollo Space Program (1967), Computers in Higher Education (1967), The World's Food Supply (1967), Underground Weapons Tests (1969), and The Next Decade in Space (1970).

In addition to these published papers, dozens of carefully prepared reports submitted through the Science Advisor to the President and his staff have not been made public. Both published and unpublished reports may influence policy decisions.

The current panels of PSAC are approximately evenly divided between subject areas related to nonmilitary and to military technologies. There are panels on air traffic control, space science, the environment, educational research and development, biological science and medicine, a national policy for science and technology, urban problems, chemicals and health, and on several similar topics, as well as panels on various military matters.

The way in which PSAC subcommittees do their work varies greatly, depending on the particular subject. Some panels have a task set by a specific request from the President for organized information and advice. Sometimes the issue has rigid time constraints. PSAC subcommittees may be called in as a fire brigade to provide timely advice in an emergency. A recent case may be cited: in September, 1970, in the wake of an airplane hijacking epidemic, the question "In what ways might modern technology be utilized to reduce the risk of further instances of air piracy?" was asked with considerable urgency. The President received prompt scientific advice. Sometimes the constraints are dominated by nontemporal factors, as for example when one considers enunciating and adopting a long-term science and technology policy for this country.

In addition to responding to direct questions put by the President, for either immediate or long-term technical advice, the PSAC has some responsibility for coordinating programs in science and technology that cross departmental lines. It sometimes occurs that an agency of the federal government doesn't appreciate fully what other agencies are doing in research and development. When the PSAC chances to recognize overlap and possible redundancy, they must make such duplication of effort clear to the White House and, more specifically, to the staff of the Bureau of Management and Budget who must prepare, on the President's behalf, a federal budget for the following year. Such duplicative efforts are often quite unequal in quality and depth. Thus, PSAC subcommittees serve in part as technical auditors. In the past two years there have been instances in which PSAC recommendations have been decisive, I believe, in terminating certain long established but apparently valueless programs, in reorienting the aims and priorities of others, and in getting new initiatives underway.

A further PSAC responsibility is to bring technical problems or newly recognized possible applications of technology to the President's attention. A member of PSAC has relatively direct access to the President, when the issue is urgent, in contrast to the tremendous difficulty scientists experienced in 1940 when trying to inform President Roosevelt that an atomic weapon could conceivably be made.

Finally, PSAC has a certain role as an in-house gadfly or devil's advocate. The more critical the questioning of the details and progress of particular programs, the more accurately and quickly the agency in question can recognize weaknesses and strive to remove them. The more thorough this critical and independent review within the executive branch, the less potential remains for embarrassment at Congressional hearings.

SCIENTIFIC ADVICE AND POLITICAL REALITY

Most of the problems associated with science and public policy are terrifically complex. Lee duBridge[1] once commented that the problems which look so simple from the outside are impossibly complex when viewed from the inside. I would support a somewhat less absolute version of this sentiment. The problems are extremely, but not impossibly, complex, and are rarely separable into strictly scientific and nonscientific aspects. Specific examples may help clarify this point.

This country has not been able to provide superior health services to its citizens. The statistical information on which this conclusion rests is readily available through the publications of the World Health Organization and other agencies.

The most significant factors responsible for the comparatively poor record must be identified if there is to be an effort to improve health care.

Chemicals might be one such factor. Chemical substances may be either harmful or beneficial to health. If inappropriate or inadequate control of such substances should be identified as an important cause of ill health in America, policy changes could be introduced. One might, for example, modify lists of prohibited or recommended pharmaceutical preparations, or the laws governing drug prescriptions, and thus conceivably improve the health of the citizens.

---

[1]President Nixon's Science Advisor, 1969-1970; President of California Institute of Technology, 1946-1969.

But suppose study should lead to the conclusion that a more statistically significant correlation exists between ill health and poverty than between ill health and exposure to harmful chemicals. What would be recommended, and to whom? A problem which at first glance may seem primarily technical may have quite a different character.

Another area where technical and nontechnical problems are thoroughly homogenized is associated with safety information on chemicals. It seems reasonable, surely, to urge chemical companies to exchange with one another information they have gained through research efforts on the toxicological properties of chemical substances. Such sharing of information would both reduce research costs and alert firms in other fields to the potential hazards of certain chemical substances. This conceivably useful change in the way chemical companies in our country do business would, however, require basic modifications in the Sherman Antitrust Act, which specifically prohibits such pooling of information. There might be a way to modify and restructure the law so that exchange of safety information would be permitted or even required. It should be possible to revise the law in a way that would allow public access to the vast store of information on the toxicological properties of chemical substances now deposited in the files of the Food and Drug Administration. A broader availability of this information could benefit all in the country.

When considering policy options on the regulation of fungicides or foreign affairs, one has to compare risks against benefits. Logically, this is the only acceptable way to proceed.

Administrative agencies, however, are sometimes established and given only half of the risk-benefit duality, and they must operate accordingly. The Food and Drug Administration, for example, has the responsibility of seeing that no toxic chemicals inadvertently reach the American public. This responsibility must be the dominant concern as they decide whether new food additives or pharmaceuticals will be permitted. Quite understandably, the administrators of the FDA are reluctant to take any risks. We may not go to them to complain if a failure to take both risks and benefits into account leads to disastrous consequences.

Has anyone determined the risk Americans are willing to accept with respect to chemical substances purposefully or inadvertently introduced into commerce or the environment? Is it zero, or is it comparable to the risks they accept on the highways, at appliance stores, and in schools?

In the years ahead we may learn to discuss both risk and benefit aspects of a policy issue in the same breath, rather than exaggerating one to the exclusion of the other. Risks are more lurid, and may be played upon effortlessly by special interests.

One Swedish environmentalist has commented on this difficulty

"All of us have an interest in keeping the environment protection debate clean. We have a strong objective argument:
Let us develop it, but let us avoid exaggeration, irrelevance,
and inaccuracy. We need the informed, not the misleading,
viewpoint. Our environment requires a clean-up. Let us hope
the same is not called for in our debates."

PROBLEMS WITH THE ADVISING PROCESS

What criticisms can be leveled against the system that exists today? Perhaps the most obvious shortcoming is that the Congress of
the United States is inadequately advised on matters pertaining to science and public policy. The Executive Branch has a near monopoly of
the formal governmental advising structure.

A Representative or Senator wanting objective and competent
scientific appraisal of the technical arguments for or against some
policy proposal has limited options. He could read the press and learn
the opinions of journalists. He could appeal for help to the overworked
staff of the Legislative Reference Service, who in turn could point him
toward appropriate articles and books, but could not undertake staff
studies. He could trust blindly in the judgments of the most vocal and
agressive university scientist volunteering his expert services. But he
could never achieve parity with the Executive Branch in capacity for
analyzing the technical subsections of complex issues.

This shortcoming could be changed relatively easily. Congress
could establish its own technical advising agency. The cost would be
low, compared with current spending for its maze of committee operations. And it could thereby put itself in a much better position for
balancing the Executive Branch on technically conditioned issues in an
informed and responsible manner.

Another criticism often heard is that undue secrecy pervades the
operations of the advising structure: meetings are not public, and only
some reports are released for general distribution. It has been proposed
recently that presidential advisors who find that their advice is ignored
or misrepresented ought to break their pledge of confidentiality and
take their case to the American people. They should publicly divulge
through the press the discrepancies between their advice and what was
subsequently formulated as national policy.

This interesting suggestion requires more careful analysis than
can be devoted to it here. My own feeling is that in extreme cases

such action might conceivably become a necessity; under normal conditions it would be an extraordinarily unsuccessful tactic for fostering more democratic government. Were the confidentiality of meetings in constant jeopardy, few would speak frankly, and the decision-making deliberations of the government would be driven underground.

The current arrangement, in which around 300 part-time advisors have placed themselves under an obligation of confidentiality, does not strike me as particularly stultifying to debate. There are tens of thousands of scientists in the country who can speak out on any issue, either as experts or as concerned but not specially qualified citizens.

But, it is commonly argued, only those on the "inside" have full access to pertinent documents and information, and hence credulity rests entirely on the side of the formal advising establishment. This opinion, however, is not well founded. Most of the facts one needs for an analysis of most issues are in the public domain, and through a little hard work and investment of time one may go through the self-education process, come to a scientific judgment, and make this known to other citizens.

There are many pressures on scientific and other sorts of advisors, both external and internal.

The external pressures come from those who are to receive the advice, or those who may be affected by it. McGeorge Bundy, while President Kennedy's Special Assistant on National Security Affairs epitomized an attitude toward scientists shared by many policy makers: "The scientist should carefully limit the occasions on which he speaks *ex cathedra* so that he is not placed in danger of losing his reputation." Of course, a scientist may never speak *ex cathedra;* scientific peers are always able to call him to task if he speaks nonsense, be it ever so technical an issue. But Bundy's implication is clear: scientists should restrict themselves rigidly to technical matters, and not attempt to influence policy or meddle in politics.

Perhaps we are now past the point where scientists claim a special infallibility, or their fellow citizens are prone to accept them as oracles.

The internal, self-generated pressures are every bit as great as those imposed from without. One must constantly face the subtle internal pressures associated with trying to preserve position. Every advisor must resist the self-limiting temptation—to avoid speaking a truth that challenges the consensus or the orthodoxy of the moment.

In resisting both internal and external pressures, one may be guided and supported by the motto, "Speak Truth to Power." The only way an advisor can keep his head is to concentrate on seeking the truth diligently and then speaking it plainly, where and when it may do some good.

THE PROSPECTS FOR ADVICE

Scientists would have a greater influence on public policy if they would trouble themselves to learn in more detail how the public business is done in Washington, and in Springfield and Chicago, and how technical information may be more effectively communicated to a non-scientific public.

Organic chemists at the University of Illinois remember when Frank Westheimer visited Urbana shortl c after publication of the Westheimer Report.[2] We asked for his reactions to the reception given the report in the press. His first comment was that, as soon as the press conference called to announce publication of the report was over, he knew that a public relations expert should have been secured. The Westheimer Report, outlining the successes of chemistry in this country in recent years and the needs of chemistry in the immediate future, was presented to the press by scientists unskilled in press conference techniques. There was no real meeting of minds between the press, who asked the wrong questions, and the scientists, who had prepared for questions that remained unasked. The report never had the public impact it might have had if the presentation to the press had been as effective as the writing.

Two years ago we had some controversy over a planned shipment of 8000 tons of obsolete nerve gas to a storage site in a remote area of Oregon. Some citizens considered the plan risky and ill-advised. Eight university scientists concerned about the matter did the required background reading and put together a position paper. They sent this statement to the President, the Surgeon General, Senators, Representatives, the Governor, and other public officials, along with some specific requests. They also called a press conference to communicate their concern to other citizens of the town and state. One of the scientists came to the press conference equipped with what I considered a silly gimmick: a photograph of a human hand, spotted with two droplets of colored water showing the approximate lethal doses of the two nerve agents that were to be shipped from Okinawa through the state of Washington to Oregon. Of course, the photographs made the first page of the newspapers, and brought the attention of the citizenry to the issue far more effectively than all of our carefully worded paragraphs analyzing the technical and legal issues involved.

Scientists having specific advising roles in the governmental advising establishment, and those without such formalized connections to individuals and agencies making and administering public policy, can learn to express more effectively the truths their specialized knowledge and intensive study lead them to recognize and formulate. Both have the same fundamental responsibility: to participate actively and honestly in the democratic process, to speak and respond, whatever the circumstances of location or position, as men sharing and willingly accepting an obligation with respect to the future.

The often posited dichotomy between insiders and outsiders, used to denote those working inside and outside of the formal advising structure is, I feel, an insignificant contrast when compared with that between insiders, who work within the framework set by history and the ideal of a participatory democracy, and the outsiders, who stand outside this common mantle of shared past and sought future.

A scientific advisor to the government and a scientific activist, working in an action group attempting to influence some public policy, have more in common than either has with a narrow academic, who considers his research specialty more significant than the public good.

There are occasions when sound technical advice is politically unacceptable. An example will make this clear. Early in the 1920's design engineers employed by Alfred Krupp started work on the next generation of German tanks, despite treaty obligations prohibiting such activity. The design effort was led by Eric Muller; the engineering was done primarily by Ferdinand Porsche and his son, designers of the Mercedes SS sports car and the Auto Union six-liter racing car. They designed many tanks, each considered ideal for a specialized land combat role, including two models 7 and 40 times heavier than their 25-ton Panthers! The tanks that were subsequently built and employed in the Second World War weren't very good. The leaders of the German tankers fighting on the eastern front recognized this promptly.   The Soviet T-34 tanks were simpler and more rugged, and they had the wide treads needed to negotiate muddy terrain.

An advising team from the German General Staff went to the front in 1941 to consider the situation. It concluded and recommended that Germany utilize captured Russian blue-prints, retool production facilities, and start turning out German-made Soviet T-34 tanks. This may have been excellent advice, but the idea that German design engineers had done an inferior job was difficult for the German political leaders to accept.   The recommendation was shelved.   Two years later the inevitable happened. The largest armor battle in history was joined at Kursk. The Soviets and the Germans each deployed about 3,000 tanks. By the end of the two-week battle, the Germans had lost 2,900 tanks and 70,000 men.

In a whole variety of circumstances it is conceivable that sound technical advice may be irrelevant; or it may be extremely apt yet politically unacceptable.   There is usually a price to pay for unjustified but staunchly-held illusions.

One scientist who exhausted himself trying to reshape public policy was Leo Szilard. At one juncture of discouragement he lamented, "There is no market for wisdom in Washington. Governmental officials are too concerned with day-to-day crises. There are too many pressures." Despite this very pessimistic pronouncement he helped form shortly thereafter a council for abolishing war which raised money to help peace candidates for public office. The $50,000 they raised in 1962 was invested in four senatorial campaigns: those of Joseph Clark in Pennsylvania, George McGovern in South Dakota, and Wayne Morse in Oregon were successful, while Stuart Hughes, running as an Independent, was defeated in Massachusetts by Edward Kennedy. In South Dakota, McGovern defeated his opponent by only 600 votes.

An activist-scientist, with the help of friends and a few contributions, did apparently make a politically significant difference. His faith was stronger and more important than his articulated pessimism.

In contrast with Szilard's view, I think there is a market for wisdom in Washington today, at least some of the time and at least on some of the issues. And one ought to make the most of it.

SUGGESTED READING

For general background, see H. Brooks, "The Government of Science", Cambridge, MIT Press, 1968, and F. von Hippel and J. Primack, "The Politics of Technology", Palo Alto, Stanford University Press, 1970. The latter work includes a well-organized summation and documentation in its second section: The Federal Science Advisory Establishment: A Handbook.

"Speak Truth to Power" was a charge given to Eighteenth Century Friends. A book with this motto as title (Philadelphia, American Friends Service Committee, 1955) develops some of the implications of the injunction.

On German tanks at the battle of Kursk, see H. Guderian, "Panzer Leader," New York, Dutton, 1952; R. M. Ogorkiewicz, "Armor: The Development of Mechanized Forces," London, Stevens and Sons, 1960; A. Werth, "Russia at War 1941-1945," New York, Dutton, 1964; W. Manchester, "The Arms of Krupp," Boston, Little, Brown, 1968.

73 74 75 76 77 9 8 7 6 5 4 3 2 1